the hip girl's guide
to homemaking

the hip girl's guide to homemaking

Decorating, Dining, and the Gratifying Pleasures of Self-Sufficiency— on a Budget!

Kate Payne

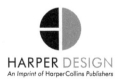

HARPER DESIGN
An Imprint of HarperCollins Publishers

HarperCollins books may be purchased for
educational, business, or sales promotional use.
For information please write: Special Markets
Department, HarperCollinsPublishers,
10 East 53rd Street, New York, NY 10022.

First published in 2011 by
Harper Design
An Imprint of HarperCollins *Publishers*
10 East 53rd Street
New York, NY 10022
Tel: (212) 207-7000
Fax: (212) 207-7654
harperdesign@harpercollins.com
www.harpercollins.com

Distributed throughout the world by
HarperCollinsPublishers
10 East 53rd Street
New York, NY 10022
Tel: (212) 207-7000
Fax: (212) 207-7654

Designed by Suet Yee Chong
Illustrations by Meredith Dawson
Calligraphy by Alison Hanks

Library of Congress Cataloging-in-
Publication Data
    Payne, Kate (Kathryn E.)
        Hip girl's guide to homemaking / Kate
    Payne. – First Edition.
        pages cm
        ISBN 978-0-06-201470-2
        1. Housekeeping. 2. Do-it-yourself work.
I. Title.
    TX321.P39 2011
    648–dc22   2010042770

Printed in the United States of America
First printing, 2011

I dedicate this book
to all the beginners out there.

Keep at it;
we all have to start somewhere.

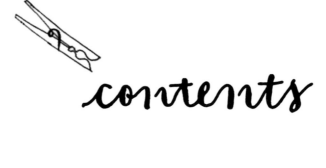

contents

PART II

Impressive Acts of Domesticity:
Do Try This at Home

PART III

Life After Restaurants

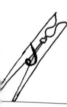

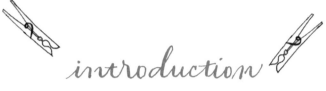

introduction

The impetus for writing this book was my manic (and true Cancerian) need to establish a comfortable home upon my arrival in New York City in the fall of 2008. I work from home, so a careless attempt at "home" just would not do, not with the chaos of big-city life lurking just on the other side of my door.

I'm not going to lie to you: most of the things I've written about here were rather daunting to me at first glance too. This book materialized from coaxing myself into and eventually reconciling with the formerly intimidating task of keeping house (while maintaining some sort of life outside the home).

I didn't learn many of these things growing up, or if I did, I blocked them out entirely. I was surely not a natural born homemaker, or even remotely good at things domestic. My mother swears we sewed together, but thoughts of my grandma's handmade blouses and slacks deeply frightened me at age thirteen, so I conveniently left that skill-sharing session off the mental record. I wasn't bad at cleaning when I was growing up, but those times I mustered up the inspiration to do it were because I was grounded or extremely broke.

As it turns out, moving to Brooklyn served as inspiration in both of the aforesaid capacities. I didn't have much money in hand (still don't) and was sequestered at home (still am), so I had to learn how to make my home a livable one out of necessity. After the house was reasonably settled, I kept going and decided to learn how to incorporate other impressive acts of domesticity into my routine. With a how-hard-can-this-be attitude and a little help from some friends who actually knew what they were doing, I discovered and cultivated a new confidence in myself as I learned these skills. You will too after you learn some of these tasks.

To use this book as a quick decorating-on-the-cheap reference, check out Part I, "Room-by-Room Guide to a Homey House, Homie." If you're wanting to read the book as a source for dredging up inspiration for the more housewifey tasks at hand, then Part II, "Impressive Acts of Domesticity: Do Try This at Home," is a fun section to peruse. Consult Part III, "Life After Restaurants," for a baby-steps introduction to your kitchen and things you might eventually do in there.

Part I provides quick and easy solutions to make your place cozier. These are steps that won't take all day or a week's pay. Check out these low-cost, creative touches to help you tap into and show off your inner artist.

Part II is the meat and potatoes of home ass-kicking, from attempting your own mending to getting happy life stains off your prized linens and cleaning with stuff you could eat (not that you actually want a baking-soda-and-vinegar cocktail). Every hip homie should get tight with his or her tool kit; after all, it's not exactly useful when you don't know how to use it.

Part III is all about impressing yourself (and others) with the gratifying pleasures of kitchen self-sufficiency; this is a first-time guide for the first-time cook, baker, home preserver, and entertainer. Regardless of the size of your kitchen, you'll learn how to make your own convenience products and not spend the few dollars you have on things you can do yourself. Most important, you'll find out how to show off your hard work by having people over to enjoy your space.

why homemaking?

Because it's cool to have a cool house. It's damn gratifying to throw down a loaf of homemade bread with your home-preserved blueberry jam. Because feeling in control in your own house does wonders for every instance when you're not under that sweet roof.

This book is for your first forays into householding tasks, both alone and with others, from college through the middle adult years. It's for all the ladies and gents who need a place to relax and rejuvenate; maybe you're single and lovin' it, or maybe you (and spouse) fit all the components of the traditional household unit yet your place (or attitude) still feels wan. No matter your station in life, you deserve a charming and inviting place to call home.

So what do you do? Do you entrust this feat to IKEA? Do you ignore it entirely? Do you think it impossible until you've found a significant other? A roommate who does dishes? Here's your guidebook, you the reluctant homemaker, charming individual, to extend the personality I know you have into the home (which I also know you have).

For the record, I'll never assume that all this stuff is easy breezy (when placed in the context of your entire life). I understand that the home feels like the never-ending chorey, and I'm a firm believer that sometimes looking the other way is the best solution.

Just remember: the house is supposed to be relaxing, and if it's your attitude toward it that's stressing you out, just change your mind. Don't think about the stack of laundry you should put away, the sweeping under the bed that never actually happens, how the plants didn't get watered. You, the house, and likely even the plants will survive. Make a list, and then schedule yourself at home to manage these things under less pressure.

housekeeping under fire

Those old-school homekeeping manuals, though handy, are a bit unwieldy in times of chaos. The only time I consult mine is when something's gone wrong: I've dyed all my whites a pretty shade of pink with an insurgent sock, or I've forgotten for the seven hundredth time on which side of the plate the napkin should be placed. Nowadays the Internet spouts at least ten answers before we can even glance over at the bookshelf, so why another book?

The digital age has its perks, don't get me wrong. But the digital age is uninspiring, to say the least. Sure, I can double-click my way to instructions for just about anything, but rarely do those instructions seek me out. You have to *want* to do these kinds of things, and you have to know how to ask the questions.

What's more, if a task seems intimidating (as most everything does for any novice), the chance that you'll give it a try is slim to none.

I hand you a book, dear reader, so you don't just bookmark these things as ideas to try someday. I think you, O busy one, can swing most of this stuff before the next time you even review your browser bookmarks.

I advocate for strength in numbers, the involvement of real friends (whom you may or may not have found through Facebook or Twitter), and the experience of hands-on knowledge. You'll learn how to throw parties on the fly, share skills or craft parties, and get people in your home for real live ways to show off your domestic accomplishments.

whose job is this anyway?

Busy working women have existed throughout time. My great-grandmother Harriet was a live-in housekeeper and nanny for a wealthy family in Michigan, leaving domestic duties in her own home to the eldest of her eight children. Grandma Mannie—Bertha Burnham, whom you'll meet periodically throughout the book—stole warm cookies from the countertop (rather than help bake them) and chased after the boys in the marshland behind their house. She remains anti-domestic.

My great-grandmother Rose, on the other hand, had the time to cook, entertain, and keep house. She baked bread weekly and imparted this (along with many other tools for domestic bliss) to her only daughter, Virginia—Grandma Jinny.

I'll not make this book about gender, because the advice in this book is as much for guys as it is for girls. Let's make this about life in general. I'm a girl, so this is obviously from my perspective, but I live with another girl, so who's supposed to do all this stuff around the house?

We've come up with a system of democratically delegating household chores based on what we each don't hate doing. I hate mopping, so she does it. She hates laundry, so I do it. This system works with roommates, romantic partners, and spouses. Giving, taking, doing more than your fair share sometimes—thus is the nature of relationships with anyone (and holds true with the home).

Whether you fit the standard mold or maybe shaped your own, roles are interchangeable in the complex, modern house. One thing it seems we all have in common, no matter what type of household we keep or background we come from: there's too much to do, and not enough time in the day to do it.

the convenience truth

How did our urgent need for convenience arise? Our prepackaged and heavily processed lifestyles have roots in a few major historical events. Here is a (really) short history: women landed the role of domesticity throughout most cultural traditions for all sorts of reasons, the handy possession of a uterus included at the top of most lists; America became a nation; a lot of things happened (i.e., household production ceased, the industrial revolution occurred, the food industry was born, wars took place, etc.).

I'll leave you to unpack each chunk of history and piece them together at your own leisure. Suffice it to say that most of our present social mores and ideas surrounding homemaking and all things domestic came from extra household income and corporate boardrooms in the postwar era. For example, the convenience food industry was born out of the need to turn profitable wartime food into postwar consumer demand (think SPAM).

The gendered history of housewifery is filled with socioeconomic and cultural land mines. So let's shift focus to address whoever is doing stuff around the house, and all the different kinds of households we see nowadays.

Phasing out convenience foods allows for smarter, healthier, and oftentimes cheaper alternatives. This is not to say that homemade food is inconvenient; after all, it's hard to determine whether or not something is convenient if you've never once tried making it for yourself. Don't worry, this book isn't about dogmatic approaches or all-or-nothing attitudes. We're all busy. We have a lot to get done in a day and usually not enough time to do it, but let's not forget how to use our common sense too.

famous last words

I have to trick myself into productivity.

I admit it; I said this. And though I'm not at all a fan of people who quote themselves, this one landed on the quote wall started at my former office. We were grant writers in tight quarters; we needed some linguistic inspiration. I think you'll find it helpful too. Here's your own little quote wall to keep with you along your way through this book.

We need a wife.

Newlywed Jed sighs as he looks at his lovely wife, Sarah. They both work full-time and find it hard to manage their dry cleaning pickup, much less eat dinner together at a reasonable hour.

We are tending [to housework and children], but few of us have the option of doing it without also holding down a job that pays real money. Home-making is moot if you're homeless. . . . Given that we have to make our own way in this big old world, it seems rude to try to make women (or men) feel guilty about neglecting the household operation.

Barbara Kingsolver reminds us that excess homemaking guilt is unreasonable in the essay "The Household Zen" from her book *High Tide in Tucson* (HarperCollins, 1995).

Just as in planting a seed and seeing it come up, there is a visible connec-tion between mixing a few ingredients and seeing the resulting product emerge. Such a relationship is genuinely straightforward. . . . When we grab a commercial product, there is, I think, a false sense of simplicity.

Annie Berthold-Bond introduces us to making our own cleaning and body care products from a few basic (and nontoxic) house-hold ingredients in her book *Better Basics for the Home: Simple Solu-tions for Less Toxic Living* (Three Rivers, 1999).

Much of the appeal of the industrial food chain is its convenience; it offers busy people a way to delegate their cooking (and food preservation) to oth-ers. . . . [A] successful local food economy implies not only a new kind of food producer, but a new kind of eater as well, one who regards finding, preparing, and preserving food as one of the pleasures of life rather than a chore.

Michael Pollan illustrates the subject of his *Omnivore's Dilemma* (Penguin, 2006) by tracing various food chains from field to table.

Don't own so much clutter that you will be relieved to see your house catch fire.

Wendell Berry telling it like it is in "Prayers and Sayings of the Mad Farmer," a poem from his book *Farming: A Handbook* (Har-court, 1970).

You can do this yourself, with your brains and your own two hands. You don't need to get it from a package. You can take charge. You can stand at the center of your own world and create something very good, from scratch.

Laura Shapiro sums up Julia Child's and Betty Friedan's messages in her book *Something from the Oven* (Viking, 2004).

Part 1

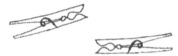

Room-by-Room
Guide to a
Homey House, Homie

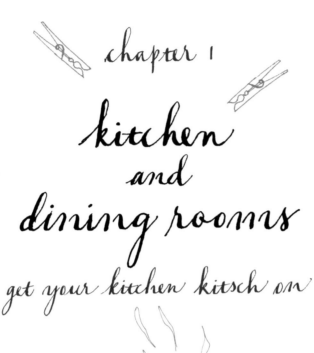

chapter 1

kitchen
and
dining rooms

get your kitchen kitsch on

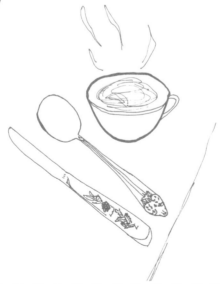

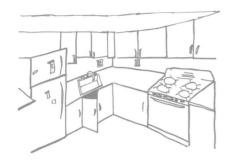

Visitors make a beeline for kitchens because it's the least awkward place to be in a stranger's house. We all have kitchens, and we all sort of know what to do in them. Couches, living rooms, and entryways, by contrast, are all places where there's nothing to do but gawk and stare at each other's kneecaps and wall décor. I'm sure this kitchen-flypaper effect has something to do also with the fact that food and the people who cook it are usually found there.

practicality meets personality

My kitchen is the least decorated room of the house. Spend a week actually using your kitchen and then tell me that certain elements of style or flair we tend to see in décor magazines and design books are not a total pain in the ass in the throes of cooking, cleaning, and eating. Be smart and decorate with your tools; make what's practical also an indicator that you have personality and a keen design sense.

We'll explore ways to populate your fridge and pantry shelves in Chapter 8, but for now, let's get the structure ready: shelves, containers, seating arrangements, and routine maintenance.

develop a relationship with your dishes

An affinity for certain everyday items might inspire you to use them more often. Breakfast at my house usually involves our Arizona state plate, the Charles and Di 1981 wedding plate I found years ago for $3 at a San Francisco stoop sale, or my 65¢ leaf-carved yellow teacup. These dishes are some of my most prized possessions (and collectively cost less than breakfast at the airport).

If sentimentality toward the things you use every day seems far-fetched, just ask yourself a few simple questions: Do you like your dishes? Do you still have that set from Target that your mom bought you as you were packing up for dorm life? They were probably on sale. Mine were hunter green and nondescript (translate: boring).

You shouldn't feel bad about placing boring, cheap dishes in the care of Goodwill or the Salvation Army, since you might buy a few of your new dishes there when you drop off the old ones. When you find a dish you like, practice the one-in-one-out rule (unless you're in straight acquisition mode) and select a dish to donate from your cabinet that garners only so-so feelings.

diversity is the spice of life

Mix-and-match dishes and silverware are functional ways for you to show off and, more important, enjoy aspects of your personality in your home. By selecting beautiful and useful pieces that go well together or that just make you happy, you're setting yourself up for home life success.

You can always go out and spend money on a fancy new set of matching dishes or silverware. But for some people that's not an option or not desirable. Instead, take to the thrift store! I can find at least one interesting drinking glass and/or teacup in any city's thrift store. The trick is to enter the store with blinders. Ignore all the weird, crappy stuff that stands out.

As you begin your dish mission, focus. Look at the items individually, not in the context of the other dull things. Sometimes it helps to write a list and keep it in your wallet, since the thrift store can be entirely overwhelming with all its tacky stuff (or sometimes with too much good stuff).

decorate with dishes

Once you've equipped your shelves with things you actually like, show 'em off! I keep big/useful/cute kitchen utensils in a vintage coffee tin on the counter because it saves space in the drawer, looks great, and places my tools within reach. Score!

Get creative with your utensil container. Look for a wide metal container like mine, a wide-bottomed glass jar, or a ceramic jar—anything that can be cleaned well (or lined) and will remain upright when a handful of utensils are inserted.

Display your teacups, people, those gorgeous, hand-selected personality pieces. Grab a few screw hooks (or S-hooks if you're hanging cups from some sort of rack) at the hardware store for about 20¢ apiece and turn the underside of a crowded cupboard into a fine (and accessible) place to stash tea settings.

decorate with food

What do you use in the kitchen every day? (Do you know yet? Don't fret if you're new to the idea.)

Our countertop staples/decorations include salt, pepper, and olive oil. We use them all the time and showcase them proudly.

put a lid on it

Mason or other glass jars from food long ago ingested are a perfect way to store new foods and condiments, since they're airtight, see-through, and much better-looking than some bland (and potentially expensive) plastic storage container.

→ *Grains.* Get them out of bulk plastic bags in your precious cupboard or pantry space and into quart-sized jars. A whole flat of these jars will run you around $14, and they're crazy useful. Or reuse jars from pickles, pasta sauce, or other large-volume liquids. We went pickle crazy last summer and ended up with ten

dish soap diluting

Save money with this unique décor idea. Tools needed: empty olive oil bottle (the fancier ones usually come in exotic, slender bottles perfect for your dish suds) and an oil pourer (the spout you'd use to pour olive oil; spend the $5 or $6 on a sturdy metal one, as opposed to the $1.99 version, and you'll be glad you did). Slender vintage bottles will also do; just be sure the pourer fits snugly and properly inside the bottle's rim.

Squirt your dish soap of choice into the clean bottle, filling it halfway. Fill the bottle up almost the rest of the way with room-temperature water, leaving an inch or two unfilled at the top of the jar. Use your hand to cover the rim completely and then invert the bottle five or six times. You want the soap to mix with the water as much as possible. This allows the dish soap to thin just enough to be expelled without clogging your decanter. Remember, you're not shaking the bottle, just practicing patience in watching the viscous dish soap mingle with water. Pop on the pourer and you're in business.

With this tip, you'll use less soap and get just-as-clean dishes. It also allows a fine opportunity to splurge on a brand of olive or other fancy-pants oil you wouldn't normally buy; dual-purpose purchasing is totally worth the extra cost in the long run.

repurposing your pickle jars like a pro

- - - - - - - - - - - - - - -

1. Start with a good wash in warm soapy water.

2. If your jar still reeks of pickles after a good washing, sprinkle some baking soda into the jar and use a damp sponge to gently scrub around the inside of the jar. Fill with water and let the baking soda solution sit overnight if necessary.

3. Remove labels by peeling off as much as you can or by (carefully) using a single-edged razor blade.

4. Use a few drops of Citra Solv on a damp washcloth to remove remaining label goo.

matching pickle jars, which turned into fine grain bins.

➥ **Spices and other dried foods.** These things keep best in the airtight environment that jars afford nicely.

➥ **Sea salt.** The one food item that should be on every countertop, easy to grab in pinches here and there. Ours is occupying a quarter-pint mason jar. Don't keep too much out or you won't use it fast enough and it'll acquire unwanted debris.

the spice rack dilemma

Whatever you do, don't rush out to a box store to buy that gigantic metal ($30 and up) spice rack that will sit large and in charge on your counter. The magnetic fridge-side ones are a little better, but generally those containers are way too large for real-life kitchen spice use. You'll end up filling the bin and then watching spices go stale before you use a quarter of them. Boo to that method.

Instead, keep your bulk-bought spices (as discussed in Chapter 8's "Bulk Binge" section) from composting in their non-biodegradable plastic bag by putting them in little glass spice jars, which can be organized by size and frequency of use. Place these jars in small pull-out trays and stack two or three trays no higher than eye level in your cabinet by using a space-saver rack, found in any store's home organization section or at the home organization mecca, the Container Store.

This method also allows you to include and incorporate the occasionally purchased plastic or glass spice containers that weren't found in the bulk area.

get your cookbooks out of the living room

Where are your cookbooks? Are they handy? I didn't think so.

Keep kitchen-specific books in or near the kitchen; you'll be likely to actually use them. I'll talk more about cookbooks in Chapter 8, but do your homework now by checking out a few classics from the library to see which instruction styles suit you best. I suggest looking through these:

- *How to Cook Everything* by Mark Bittman
- *The Joy of Cooking* by Irma Rombauer
- *On Food and Cooking: The Science and Lore of the Kitchen* by Harold McGee

clothespins

I don't mind telling you with certainty that clothespins will change your life. Clothespins are the most essential item in my homekeeping. During a long stay when I helped my mom recover from surgery, she drove me to three stores in icky winter weather to find clothespins, since I was to be her homekeeping housemate.

Hip Trick

You can write on any glass jar or container with a Sharpie marker—and easily remove the writing with a dab of rubbing alcohol!

five things to do with clothespins in the kitchen

1. Say good-bye to chip clips, those ugly plastic things that break under pressure. It seems there are never enough of these clips to cover all the things that need cinching, and they come in obnoxious colors to boot.

2. Hang single-page recipes above your workspace. Or clip a group of pages in a cookbook to keep it open to the page in use.

3. Affix your gloves to a place near the sink. Mine are clipped to the watering pail stashed above our sink.

4. Pin your apron(s) to one of the less-used drawer handles for handy access.

5. Hang still-drying Ziplocs on various objects in your kitchen (if you run out of room on the drying rack).

make arrangements: sitting down with your food

Where you sit and where guests sit is hopefully one and the same place. I advocate for a small kitchen table centrally located in the kitchen if possible. Most home builders and designers understand the fundamental principle of eating in or near where the food is made. Maybe you're blessed with a grown-up dining room just off the kitchen. I'm not, but that hasn't stopped me from hosting a fourteen-person seated dinner. More to come in Chapter 10 on how I moved my futon into the hallway to accommodate a makeshift extended table for fourteen.

For now, let's focus on you having a seat.

the kitchen table

It's time to ritualize the process of sitting down with your food (and not at your computer desk). Here's where the kitchen table comes in handy.

Of the staple furniture pieces, the kitchen table is perhaps one of the toughest pieces to come by on the cheap. I inherited my 1950s-style leather-topped four-seater from friends who upped their family size. Refer to the "Shopping and Scavenging Like a Pro" section in Chapter 2 for ideas on how to find "the one" without going broke.

Most important, hold out for the right one,

and don't be hasty. A card or fold-up table decked out with a nice tablecloth is an excellent interim piece (and a staple in the kind of entertaining done in Chapter 10) until you meet your table soul mate. Whatever you use as a table, just be sure your legs will fit underneath it without disturbing the setup.

If a table and chair or two do not fit in your kitchen, then place your setup as near your kitchen as possible. Proximity breeds regularity. (And besides, who wants to schlep a fine meal's accoutrements through your bedroom, bathroom, and/or laundry room?)

If you're carving out a dining area from a larger room, try to keep this area as uncluttered as possible in terms of décor. The table is a prominent enough feature, so regardless of its individual style, focus attention there rather than incorporating stuff on the walls or loading up shelving. Anchoring your table to a free wall (so it juts out lengthwise) will help set the tone for turning this area into an eating and sitting area versus a cluttered corner where you stuck a table and some chairs.

While it may be chic, a rug underneath the kitchen or dining room table is counterproductive to cleaning efforts. Stuff spills under the table all the time; the last thing you need is to rack up dry cleaning bills from the act of using your table properly. If you must have a rug, try to stick with an easily spot-treated or machine-washable one.

chairs

You can never have too many. We pick them up off the side of the road whenever we find a sturdy one. A layer of paint or wood glue usually does wonders for an unfortunately painted or wobbly chair. When scavenging for additional seating, pay close attention to the underlying design. Your chair collection doesn't have to match, but an ultramodern find will stand out in the wrong kind of way if the rest of your décor is vintage, so try to snag ones that will go together or play off one another.

Don't bother with chairs that need extensive work to make them usable, like ones with broken legs or missing seats, unless you're into those types of fixer-upper projects.

Most important consideration in chair choice: comfort. You'll never sit at your table if the chairs aren't sturdy and reasonably comfortable. Try dressing up hard wooden chairs with simple, washable seat cushions. No need to buy anything fancy; a thin pillow is essentially a seat cushion.

keep it clean

A space for eating doesn't do you much good if it's covered with dishes from last Tuesday, knickknacks, stacks of paper, utility bills, three months' worth of newspapers, business cards for people you'll never call . . . you get the point. The first part of starting a ritual begins with how you practice establishing rules.

Our table backs up with newspapers still, but that stack of out-of-date *New York Times* sections inhabits the third, usually unoccupied, seat.

skirting the issue

Real-deal linens add color, style, and old-school flair to your home. If you have a less-than-enchanting kitchen table for the time being, a tablecloth instantly transforms and inspires. Cloth napkins are my first choice for a quick and easy way to add character to your pad. Yes, I know, you have to wash these things, but you also have to wash your underwear, and I don't hear you complaining about that.

tablecloths

When I was on a trip home a few years ago, my mom passed along two family heirlooms: lace tablecloths. Unfurling Great-Grandma Rose's long lace tablecloth in my apartment, I discovered the family tree of food stains, dating back to when I was little and further back to before my dad ever sat at the table.

Finding everyday tablecloths can be a challenge. When purchased new at a big-box store, they're either vinyl or end up looking like a stiff, bland banquet tablecloth. The small, square, pretty tablecloths are real diamonds in the rough, and they're almost exclusively vintage (and can include other people's happy life stains).

Take to thrift and antiques stores, and read on for tips on finding cool linens on the cheap. As you're hunting around for cute vintage tablecloths, expect to pay at least $10, but don't buy anything over $25 (unless you *have* to have it). You're eating off this thing; someone might spill wine or olive oil on it.

I do love my old tablecloths and will continue to buy them with minor stains or small holes. Most of the time these flaws are not easily noticeable, and other times a simple shift of a place mat, visit from the needle-and-thread fairy, or strategically placed vase will draw attention elsewhere.

place mats

Consider these a protection zone for your linens. They can be cool-looking, not just woven or gingham patterns that remind

13

you of eating cereal and gazing into space throughout your childhood. Our charming vinyl numbers relieve me of my inner midwestern tendencies (which make stain prevention my focus rather than allowing me to relax and enjoy suppertime and company). I no longer fret in secret about how that slosh of oily vinaigrette is going to be a royal pain in the ass, if not impossible, to remove from our white frilly tablecloth.

I make it a habit to look at the linen section of any thrift store I enter because treasures do exist. Linen sections will trick you. I scored our quirky elk and coral reef place mats at a Salvation Army hanging among godawful things. Once removed from the context of overused twin bedsheets and matching ugly shams doubled over on hangers, these place mats' charm grew exponentially.

Now, thanks to that $3.99 purchase, I am no longer that crazy grandma figure who sets out in a frenzy to cover the whole house in plastic.

napkins

I've learned to avoid the siren song of pastel or, God forbid, white napkins because whoever deemed them appropriate for regular table use must have been on a diet consisting solely of cereal and lunch meat. Cooking done in our household involves butter or olive oil, both of which are light-colored napkins' fatal enemies.

Look for dark-hued, pretty patterns. The cool thing about patterns (as opposed to solid colors) is how they camouflage grease stains and spots. You get stylish table settings without spending hours in the laundry room (or hunkered over the bathtub) spot-treating and hand-washing a friggin' napkin.

I chanced upon a set of eight navy blue, rose-patterned napkins at Goodwill. This impromptu linen excursion continued to pay off when I dug deeper into the nondescript cardboard box piled high with excess linens (those that had yet to, and might never, make it to hangers) when I spotted a set of six brown West Elm napkins with a single-leaf design. Though the brown set isn't my everyday style, it can never hurt to have extra napkins on hand to mix and match for dinner parties or for times when your laundry schedule is a little behind.

What's more, two bundles of napkins, fourteen in total, cost me a grand total of $4.31.

finding chic linens on the cheap

- ⇢ Thrift stores such as the Salvation Army, Goodwill, or Savers are your best bet for cheap and possibly vintage linens. However, be prepared for disastrous piles of ugly stuff. There are diamonds in the rough; they're just usually at the bottom of that box in the corner.

- ⇢ Antiques stores frequently have an array of grandma-inspired tablecloths. Napkins are a little iffy since it seems like all that gets planted in these places are the white linen, tea napkin sets, and clearly, I vote no on light-colored linens for sanity purposes.

- ⇢ Etsy. I know you know about this website, but I'll bet you haven't thought to buy vintage napkins here. You'll also find contemporary hand-stitched and embroidered linens, and (big plus) the vendors actually mail them to you.

- ⇢ Many cities have a citywide garage sale or big charity

garage sale of some sort where you pay by the pound for what is mostly antique and vintage stuff. Bring a cart and be prepared to fight for that perfect flowery tablecloth, though. All manners and etiquette are usually checked at the door with your coat when hitting up these seasoned-shopper conventions.

↦ Fabric stores (gasp). See the DIY napkin or tablecloth project in Chapter 6. C'mon, it's just a square piece of fabric—how hard can this be?

taking stock:
pantry closets or cupboards

Okay, let's get you prepared for Chapter 8. Walk over to your pantry closet or cupboard (or both) and look inside. Just like in yoga breathing exercises, take note of the status quo without attempting to change anything at first. Are your food items stacked precariously? Are things composting on the bottom, things you've moved in and out of numerous apartments or houses? Are you instantly able to locate and discern all types of foods: pastas, cereals, canned foods, dry goods, cookies? If this takes more than a minute of your time, read on.

sort and dispose

Add some method to your madness by doing a big ol' pantry inventory at least once a year. Any season is great for this, especially spring (think spring cleaning), when a new season of stocking up starts (more on that in Chapter 9). Don't be intimidated by this; you'll feel much better after it's done. It's an easy four-step process:

1. Pull everything out. Wipe out your cabinet shelves when the coast is clear in there; excess crumbs are an invitation for pests to visit and snack from your pantry, gross.

2. Investigate labels and expiration dates. If you don't see one but you remember moving the item at least twice, that's an automatic throw-away. Five-year-old pasta, hmm? An alternative to just pitching stuff that's marginally fresh is to set it out on the counter and use it up in the next week. There's a bit of my Depression-era granny in me, since usually I'd rather eat stale chips than throw them out. To this step, I say to each their own.

3. Now is also a good time to take note of and/or rid your pantry of food items that contain things you don't particularly want to eat, such as heavily processed foods with more than 2-inch-long lists of ingredients, or foods that contain ingredients a ten-year-old couldn't pronounce. If you feel guilty about throwing these things away, then figure out how to give them away.

4. When putting your food items back in the cabinet, group like objects. Stack soups, beans, and other cans so you can read the labels. Put things you don't use often in the back. Utilize an inexpensive space-saver rack to stack things and double your

considering ditching the microwave?

They take up valuable countertop real estate; they change the molecular structure of food in order to heat it up from the water stored within foods (which is the opposite of conventional heating methods that go from the outside in); they decrease the availability of certain nutrients in foods.

Swap it out for a good convection or toaster oven (and then you can get rid of the clunky toaster, too). We use ours to heat up leftovers, melt butter for baking, and, of course, make toast.

pantry space. Small kitchens provide plenty of opportunities for creative stashing; my favorite pantry method involves external shelving.

reuse on the run

We all know by now that popping a plastic container of leftovers into the microwave isn't a good idea because the heat increases the transfer of plastic particles into the food you're about to eat.

We made the switch from plastic to glass storage containers via a birthday gift from my future mother-in-law. (I'm glazing over the fact that I've somehow become someone excited about storage containers as a result.)

I adore my Pyrex-brand, multi-sized set because the bowls double as classy serving dishes for salsa or other treats during parties, you can write on them with a Sharpie (now that you're hip to the rubbing-alcohol trick), and they are safe for storing acidic, fatty, and salty foods without leaching plasticizers into your food.

a life less plastic

Using less plastic in the kitchen is something we decided is best for us (and the family we are hoping to have in the future). We still buy plastic wrap, but we always get the brands (such as Glad Cling Wrap, which is made of polyethylene) that do not contain the chemicals in plastics (phthalates or DEHA) that leach into foods whether you're heating them or not. The Washington Toxics Coalition advises against storing food in plastic containers when possible because it's hard to know what's in the variety of tubs and containers out there.

Plastic things you buy marked with a 1 inside the little re-cycle arrows are designed to be single-use. You might think you're being thrifty by reusing that deli-bought water bottle or plastic tray, but they can harbor bacteria if not cleaned (and dried) thoroughly, and using it more than a few times can de-grade the plastic, causing it to leach into whatever you're eating or drinking. No thanks. Switch to a metal water bottle to refill on the run.

I like the catchy mantra from the authors of *Slow Death by Rubber Duck* to help you remember which plastics are safe to buy and eat from: "4, 5, 1 and 2; all the rest are bad for you."

chrome wire shelving racks

The movable and customizable pantry! I adore these industrial wire racks (not, of course, for their inherent charm; they're pretty sterile and nondescript when empty). They're super-sturdy (most hold up to six hundred pounds) and provide an excellent oppor-tunity to decorate with practical items.

Load up shelving like this with jars of dry goods, cookbooks, kitchen linens, and large pots or appliances, and free up valu-able real estate on your countertop or in cupboards and draw-

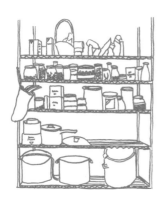

ers. These racks are also great for use with S-hooks, to hang large utensils, tea or coffee cups, and utilize all available space.

Where to put this metal skeleton? Well, rarely do you have an available wall in the kitchen (and if you do, your kitchen table should be there), so posi-tion your shelving as a means of creating depth. If you have a studio apartment, add it perpendicularly to a wall to create the illusion of separation between the kitchen area and the rest of your room. Or place it strategically (i.e., as close as possible to the kitchen) if you're working in a shoebox kitchen.

Though you don't have to spend a ton of money on a shelf like this, if there's one thing you do spend money on in setting up your kitchen space, let it be this.

Always check Craigslist first. Restaurants close and people move, so these racks are always available used. The racks are not at all difficult to disassemble, but if it's going to be an ordeal to get a used rack home in pieces, then scope out the following options for a delivered, in-box version.

- Kitchen supply stores
- Office supply stores
- Hardware stores

We actually found our rack left out by the side of the road for the trash pickup. Keep your eyes peeled; anything is possible.

If you're ordering or buying a new one, you'll likely be buying a starter unit that comes with four to six shelves, four column posts, and four wheels or stationary feet. The shelves come in a few different, standard sizes, so you can always buy extra shelves or other components later (next paycheck).

deck the walls

All that's left in your kickin' kitchen décor preparations are the walls. I've saved this area for last for a few reasons:

- Structural pieces like kitchen tables or wire racks must be in place before you know where you have free wall space.
- You are building a theme into your collection of dishes, tools, containers, and kitchen supplies (yes, even "useful" is a theme), so you'll want to pick wall hangings that feel right with your stuff.

My favorite wall hanging in any kitchen is a chalkboard, multifunctional and good for love notes, grocery lists, visitor guestbooking, or vocabulary words of the day. If you're not lucky enough to have a chalkboard wall (or if the space is too small to reasonably paint a chunk of the wall black and leave chalk next to it), hang a small, framed one. It works like a charm.

quick chic:
five kitchen décor dos and don'ts

DO

1. Buy vintage, mix-and-match cabinet and drawer pulls to distract kitchen visitors from your less-than-desirable cabinetry. Lucky scavengers might find them cheap at flea markets and antiques stores. I hunted ours down online for about $6 apiece.
2. Double the function of cute bowls by storing fruit, vegetables, nuts, or salt and pepper on your countertop. It's a win-win: show off pretty dishware and make your food accessible.
3. Buy a mountable magnetic strip to hang your knives on a small area of wall space, preferably near the

countertop, and kick that space-eating wood block to the curb.

4. Take the opportunity to hang a lacy curtain or cute fabric where you have open shelving or missing doors; it also cuts down on cooking splashes and dust settling on your dishes.

5. Stack once-in-a-while appliances and pretty cookware atop cabinets or on the fridge to leave room for your everyday items.

DON'T

1. Buy knobs or drawer pulls that don't fit the style of your kitchen (even if they're really cheap). A brushed metal set will look silly on your 1940s- or 1980s-style kitchen cabinetry.

2. Hang things where you will knock them over all the time or where you can't reach them.

3. Store knives in your countertop utensil jar. High utensil traffic will dull the blades faster.

4. Place your open-shelving curtain or cloth in a major use area because extracting items from that shelf will be annoying. If this must be the case, then be sure to use a mini-curtain rod and a fabric that slides easily.

5. Stack things so obscurely that you can't find them or where it's an ordeal to get them down (e.g., you need to haul out the ladder to get your Cuisinart).

dish duty 101:
the never-ending chorey

There's no way around it. The happy home life leaves a trail of dishes in its wake. If you're not down with dish doing, there's an appliance for you: the dishwasher. You decide. Either that's where you spend what's left of your paycheck, or start looking at doing dishes my way.

My dishes are a cathartic gateway to unlocking whatever task is at hand. The more dishes I do, the more productivity credits I garner. This may seem dramatic, but it applies to any task on your list, especially those unrelated to the kitchen. Think about it: a form of procrastination that leaves you with a clean cabinet of dishes is a real win-win situation. Your dishes will like this idea, your dinner-at-home success rate will rise, and you'll ease into the idea of productivity one clean fork at a time.

down-and-dirty dish-doing accoutrements

➻ *Gloves.* A pair of pretty and functional dish gloves can do wonders for inspiring you to take on those daunting dishes. Make sure they're accessible, though, and not crammed in a drawer underneath your prized array of rubber bands, takeout menus, and packets of spare Christmas lightbulbs. I like the Casabella brand because they're (a) hot pink, (b) thick latex with a flocked lining, meaning they last a long time and help you work with high-temperature water (like when you attempt canning and preserving in Chapter 9) and (c) water-stop designed (folded over at top) because no one enjoys getting dish slosh inside their gloves, eeewww.

23

- *Shimmy while you shammy.* Doing dishes is an excellent time to catch up on podcasts, radio news shows, or other audio media. The kitchen sink is not unlike the shower, so go ahead, belt out the lyrics to your favorite Patty Griffin album. I think dishes like being serenaded.
- *Stuck on flour sack.* Invest in dish towels you actually like. Unlike with tablecloths and napkins, it's rare that I find a used dish towel, vintage or thrift, that I like. I'm partial to the luxury of flour sack, but when it comes to vintage, either it's gone threadbare and fallen apart in Grandma's kitchen or she's still using it. Buy a pack of these towels new, four for $10 at the most. They're absorbent and soft on the hands, and they usually come in plain white or solid colors that you might (at some point down the line) embroider to personalize (or gift).

no dishwasher?

My favorite method for dishwasherless living is dish-tub washing. The dish-tub method is my pretend pioneer lady throwback—not to mention the most efficient hand-wash method—except I don't have to pitch used water off the porch when finished. I can also hear the radio better from the kitchen when the water isn't running.

Step 1: Fill a dish-tub-like object (e.g., a stock pot or a large mixing bowl) with hot water and a few squirts of undiluted dish soap. Use this tub/water combo to immerse dishes (if they'll fit) or just to refresh the sponge before you soap up each dish. After each dish is sufficiently sudsed, set them on the counter somewhere next to the sink in preparation for the rinse bath. Try to keep your suds bath relatively clean by scraping food remnants into the trash before plopping plates in the water, or dumping out presoak water from cups or bowls before you dunk them in the suds.

Step 2: Once all your dishes have been sudsed, pitch out the soapy water and rinse the container or dish tub, filling it with hot or warm water for the rinse cycle. When you're dipping dishes in the rinse tub, be sure to create a little friction—that is, give the dish a good slosh during the dunk—so that soapsuds don't cling to the dish as you pull it out of the water. Alternatively, if using a smaller improvised tub, use it to rinse silverware only and run the rest under the hot tap to rinse.

If we were really fancy, we'd have two rinses, one warm and one cold, but I get lazy and tired of standing at the sink. One rinse will do for me.

When I'm feeling particularly uninspired by the relentless daily mound of dishes, I adopt a classic Garrison Keillor–inspired approach: *it could be worse.* I think about all the people in other countries who have access to only use a fraction of the water we use here in the United States, and feel immediately grateful that I didn't have to carry home my day's water supply on my head or boil every drop of my water before using it.

resources

books

- *Slow Death by Rubber Duck* by Rick Smith and Bruce Lourie.
- *Clean and Green* by Annie Berthold-Bond. *A thorough guide to eco-friendly home set-ups.*

web

- etsy.com
  Amazing homemade items for the house.
- fishseddy.com
  Dinnerware, flatware, glassware and more!
- theimprovisedlife.com
  Loads of homemaking and household management info.

chapter 2

living areas

master sitting

without musical chairs

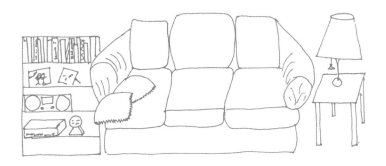

One day while walking to the subway stop with a friend, she offhandedly mentioned that she's waiting until Mr. Right shuffles in off the prairie before she'll invest any effort in a happy home life. I picked up my jaw, followed her into the train station, and pretended to take it in stride.

Let's remember, I'm a Cancerian home goddess. For all you astrology-phobes out there, that just means I nest well. For all my time dancing around the living room to Beyoncé's "Single Ladies," I've yet to hold off making a house a home. Who cares what your situation is? Whether you have roommates, occupy a super-tiny studio space, or live with a partner/spouse with opposite or no taste at all, you should always care about your home.

Just because you haven't figured out that sandpit called the "rest of your life" doesn't mean you can't have a sweet and warm place to call home for now. Treating your house like a hotel is a bummer. So let's try to figure out some ways to do real-life living in your place—by both structural and simple homey home solutions. Let me pull down the rolling map atop the chalkboard and get my pointer out.

what's in a name?

Guess what you're supposed to do in the living room? Live! Well, technically, I suppose the living room is for show—fancy pillows and uncomfortable furniture included—and "real life" happens in the family room or den. Whatever. I have one big room. I get one shot at a living- and entertaining-oriented space. I'm going to go ahead and assume you're in the same situation.

Many of us treat our furniture like decorations. We labor over getting monster-sized couches, complicated chairs, and flat-pack

IKEA furniture accompanied by not-as-easy-as-it-looks illustrated directions for assembly. These items only seem to produce dust and stubbed toes rather than that cozy home effect. Since you probably only get one area to work with, how can we make it a place where both you and guests feel at home?

the method:
distract and delight

Let's face it, your shitty apartment is not how you define yourself. If that were the case for me, I'd be ancient and falling apart. And let's also be clear: for the millions of us renting apartments and houses out there, our home design palettes are fundamentally limited (read: flawed), and we are not going to be the ones to fix them.

My house was built in 1892. I don't have doors on all the cabinets in my kitchen. My countertop, yellow Formica with faux silver trim, makes me feel like a failure if I pay it any mind. My range sits in the original cooking fireplace for the whole brownstone, dating back to when the servants' quarters were our ground-floor apartment, and the enclave has been thoughtfully painted fire engine red.

My linoleum kitchen floor, new upon our move-in a year ago, sports wear trenches and creases where plywood plank seams threaten to swallow us into the basement. No amount of paint and scrubbing will turn my house into one like those featured in do-it-yourself design magazines or HGTV budget-friendly apartment rehab shows.

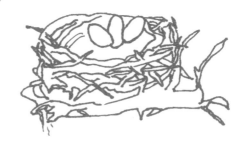

For all the flaws, there are a few

rather charming features that I play it up like it's no one's business: the original parquet flooring and intricate crown molding, which are still intact. The rest is up to my décor and style, distracting people from the house's shortcomings and delighting them with vivid colors and fun textures.

design and décor for beginners (like me)

I must make a confession. It never occurred to me to open a home décor or design manual before now, as I try to put my style—one that captures visitors' hearts—into words. After looking into it, though, it turns out that there are tons of resources out there for those without an innate sense of style and spatial relations, or for those of us lacking the ability to competently discuss it.

Living rooms are a dime a dozen. Shapes, sizes, and situations all vary, but one thing is common to all: you need to set up a place for at least two people to sit, facing each other. You can't have a conversation when you're both facing the same way (toward a television).

I'm not going to pretend that I know your unique furniture conditions, such as room shape and size, or personal habits, so I won't prescribe individual solutions here. That's what *Apartment Therapy* or HGTV is for. You can also check out the "Resources" section at the end of this chapter for shopping tips, books, and blogs that might help you with major structural or design-oriented matters. My advice serves to generally help you adjust your home with small steps.

the three r's:
reclaim, repurpose, revamp

Since living rooms are all about sitting, let's use the couch as the canvas for examples of putting these handy methods into practice. Surely you'll recognize this predicament: the grown-up couch versus the college futon—when and how to make the switch? Use your budget or desired level of involvement as a guide on this. One thing is for sure: you'll be inviting a pal over to help you put that metal-framed black futon on the curb.

RECLAIM. Post your ugly futon on Craigslist, under either "Free Stuff" or "For Sale" (depending on how much wear and tear your college years expended upon it). Craigslist is my favorite tool for furniture ridding and replacing on the cheap. There's someone out there who wants what you no longer want, and vice versa; your perfect couch dreams just might be answered through on-line classifieds. When it's time to pick out a new piece, do some hunting through gently used options before braving the IKEA maze.

REPURPOSE. Create a couch effect from things that are not normally considered couchy. Check out operations like Habitat for Humanity ReStores to purchase reclaimed items—components and materials that are salvaged from renovations and demolitions. You might find all the windowpanes you've ever dreamed of, an old church pew, or a theater row. (I don't recommend sitting on the windowpanes, though!)

REVAMP. If your budget begs to differ with your couch evolution goals, you can compromise with a grown-up futon. Swap your old one for a wood-framed futon and dress it up with a simple, elegant slipcover

31

(a roughly $40 purchase from any big-box home store). Another option is to purchase a basic coverlet, like the subtly patterned ones featured at Urban Outfitters, and tuck it snugly around your futon. Both coverlet and slipcover are easily thrown in the washing machine, too. If you're stuck with a futon, at least you get the consolation prize of still being able to accommodate sleepover guests, for those of us sans spare bedrooms.

have a seat:
living room lowdown

Does your living room encourage life forms to take a load off? Is the act of sitting down in your living room a natural process? Or would you cram yourself into a middle seat on the subway— between occupied end seats—before sitting anywhere in your house besides your bed?

Let's get touchy-feely for a minute. If we were doing a scientific experiment, this would determine your control group.

Step 1: Walk into your living room.

Step 2: Look around. Where can you sit? Couch, chair, floor?

Step 3: Note any obstructions to happy sitting, such as coats, newspapers, or (gasp) dirty dishes.

Step 4: Once sitting, note the view—a wall, table, window.

This is a great time for a flow chart! Everyone's situation will be slightly different, and each course of action somewhat specialized. Your goal is to facilitate a welcoming sitting atmosphere. There are two quick ways to get that process started:

32

1. Set furniture up so that people are facing each other.
2. Put your TV on the curb (or hide it).

If you would like a refresher on what people did before televisions became the focal part of our living rooms (and lives), pick up any Victorian novel. Those industrious folks had a lot of time on their hands (they had servants), so they perfected the art of self-improvement, entertaining, and hosting. I suggest Tolstoy's *Anna Karenina* or Jane Austen's *Pride and Prejudice* to get you going.

boob tube camouflage

The TV debate is a real biggie. If you are fine with establishing an altar to TV, then skip this section for now. Otherwise, forget the usual self-righteousness that comes along with the anti-television crowd; let's focus on the fact that it's an eyesore, plain and simple. Who wants a massive flat-screen as the centerpiece of their living area? Or a rotund dinosaur perched in the corner of the room?

You may not have final say on what happens in your living room if you live with roommates, your girlfriend/boyfriend, or a spouse, but all hope is not lost.

- An obvious first choice for hiding that unsightly screen is a special cabinet or shelving unit that gives your TV a top-secret double life, making it disappear into a wall or slide down inside a hidden drawer. But, really, who has that kind of thing, or an extra $3,000 to spare on furniture? You're lucky if you've made the upgrade from a garage-sized boxy CRT television to a flat-screen, or so I hear.

33

- Investigate the vintage furniture circuit described later in this chapter and you might find a cool-looking, potentially affordable armoire to tuck that TV out of sight. A friend of mine's husband is an industrial designer and he transformed their TV stand into a real piece of art. It's the same sort of tactic as the distract-and-delight method: absorb the TV into the larger art of the stand.
- Consider resting a lightweight piece of artwork against your TV when you're not watching it. Not having enough wall space might actually help solve the TV problem, too.

bright lights, fancy lamp

You already know that localized lighting is where it's at. There are a number of ways to infuse your living room (and other areas of the house) with fancy lighting. Track lighting is likely out of the question (it involves probing around in the ceiling, going to IKEA, and/or following directions that may or may not give guidance). If you're not up for a rewiring project or couldn't afford that antique chandelier in the first place, make your own fancy lamp out of stuff you have lying around the house.

DIY lights localization project essential tools:

- A (preferably) metal basket-like object
- A drop-hanging light cord, usually about $4
- A compact fluorescent bulb
- Two to four clothespins
- One large sheet or multiple smaller sheets of pretty

paper (try wrapping paper, wallpaper, fancy stationery store paper, or even a piece of pretty cloth)

I advise using only compact fluorescent bulbs since they don't get as hot as regular, energy-gobbling incandescents; you don't want to set your pretty paper or guests on fire.

This project can go in two different directions:

↪ **Objectify.** Suspend the lightbulb in the middle of a show-off-worthy object, like a pretty birdcage. Wrapping and looping the lightbulb cord around the top of the object is an easy, hardware-free way to suspend the bulb evenly in the middle. Hang your new object lamp or place it strategically on a shelf. Learn more about the art of hanging things from the ceiling in Chapter 7. *Note: If you're setting your crafty lamp on a shelf, make sure your lit bulb is not resting against any part of the object.*

↪ **Cover-craft.** If you're using a mundane metal object, fancy it up with pretty paper or cloth. I'm using a hanging vegetable basket as an example of a hangable metal object (something like it is always available at the thrift store), but you can use any circular or square metal object (like a filing bin for the desktop). Drop the lightbulb and cord down through the middle and either suspend them from one of the basket tiers or just set them in the basket. Wrap your cloth or paper around the rack and secure it with the clothespins. I would not leave this lamp setup on when you're not home, but you wouldn't do that anyway, would you? The electric bill isn't paid by fairies!

35

safe disposal of compact fluorescent bulbs

Never throw spent compact fluorescent bulbs in the regular garbage. They contain mercury, which will end up in our groundwater if the bulbs are not disposed of properly. Some retail and hardware stores allow you to drop off used bulbs for safe disposal. Learn about the many ways to get rid of household hazardous waste in the "Resources" section of Chapter 5.

now, test your work

Invite a friend (roommate, spouse) to sit down with you in your living room. Make coffee or tea and see if it feels natural to be sitting there. If possible, select someone who doesn't know how odd it might feel to be sitting in your house. We are creatures of routine, so someone who is used to viewing your house as a drive-through might not realize its new comfort right off the bat. For best results, repeat this test as many times as possible.

This also serves as a practice for self-sufficiency: you made something yourself, to be consumed by yourself (and others).

Explore Chapter 10 for other ideas for getting test sitters into your space, including hosting a book group, tea party, or another event to bring other humans into your space and practice using your furniture and lighting.

love your stuff

Home swag, knickknacks, and curios are all highly personal matters. If you must have them, it's key to factor them into larger design schemes. My beloved won't part with a pair of amber-colored glass mushrooms. I can't stand the things, but I love *her*, so I've compromised on allowing them to be displayed in our bedroom (a little-visited area of the house) in the corner of the windowsill. The outside glare hits them in the early afternoon, making them almost pretty, plus they sort of coordinate with the teardrop-shaped turquoise glass vase that we brought home from Oaxaca and which hangs in that same window.

I'm not an interior designer, nor a home décor specialist. I just like pretty things. I like to surround myself with things that make me happy. That's it! As our old pal William Morris said, "Have nothing in your house that you do not know to be useful or believe to be beautiful." If something's beautiful to you, find a way to make it work.

Our house is a museum of enchantments. My style translates to: if it's old, I'm all over it. So I've given prominent placement to our living room swag (items that elsewhere would be gathering dust). Obviously, you should use your favorite things. But to give you a feel for what I'm describing, here are a few of mine proudly on display:

- Typewriters (five in total)
- Cameras (at least twelve)
- Books (I've lost track)
- One vintage washboard
- A few old-timey soda and milk crates

shopping and scavenging like a pro

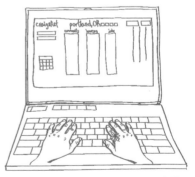

- **Craigslist** is where I look first for furniture and other major purchases. I don't buy these things new because I can't afford them. Who'd have thought you could go to one website to find a job, an apartment, and cheap furniture?

37

- **Flea markets and citywide garage sale events** are iffy but have a lot of potential. Notice the clientele: old people (good) or hip, young people like yourself (bad). Don't get me wrong, there's nothing bad about hipster flea markets, but you're not going to get an exceptionally good deal on furniture or major pieces at these types of events. They've already done the sorting through crappy furniture to find the antique-y, cute pieces for you, hence you'll pay a premium. Try to home in on vendors who specialize in certain things and then buy other things from them—that is, look for kitchenware or curios from vendors who primarily offer linens or clothing, and vice versa; that's where the deals lie. Don't be afraid to offer a lower price. The worst a vendor might say is no, and there's no harm done.
- **Thrift stores** have a needle-in-a-haystack nature to them; everyone who walks into one must hone their vision. Thrift shoppers must train the eye to find that one cute thing among the many un-cute things piled up everywhere. Rarely do I leave a thrift store, though, without some sort of prize for my scavenging efforts. Some stores will be more stocked and/or picked over than others depending on location and the neighborhoods that feed them and which have access to shopping in them.
- **Estate sales** are usually advertised in the newspaper or by signs hung around a neighborhood. Estate sales are usually coordinated by a company hired by a family who needs to sell the property (and its contents) after an elderly loved one passes away. It might

sound creepy to be rummaging through evidence of unknown years of strangers' lives, but you can think of how you'll give their belongings a lifetime of new memories. I've found great deals on vintage kitchenware, canning jars, linens, books, and excellent collage materials (old sheet music, newspapers from ye olden days, 1950s magazines with funny ads) at estate sales.

➼ **Anthropologie's sale room** is every scavenger's dream when you need something new. Items are all unused and gorgeous. There are real bargains to be found here.

➼ **Curbside trash** should not be underestimated. What's that expression? One man's trash is another man's treasure? People throw things out for all kinds of reasons, and many times it's because they just don't want the item (or no longer have room for it). You can pick up perfectly good things awaiting new homes. Finding an antique washboard on my way home—one that vendors at the local hipster flea market would sell for at least $75—gave added purpose to a baby-blue painted wooden chair we found on the curb weeks prior, two prizes that complement each other nicely!

another roadside attraction: decorating with found objects

My affinity for roadside trash really pays off in the home department. It's in my genes. Grandma Mannie got her scavenging savvy growing up in the Midwest during the Depression; hunting through trash bins behind grocery stores was not uncommon during those hard years for her and her seven brothers and sisters. Now, with no need for such drastic scavenging measures, my gram hunts around for cool furnishings that people leave out for trash. We chat about major scores every couple weeks over the phone; I giggled the other day when she told me how she leaned into the dumpster behind her apartment to snag the cute (and perfectly good) wooden magazine rack someone had pitched.

Wooden objects are common, and my favorite kind of roadside find. Old pieces of wood tell stories about the past, and in turn tell stories about your home to visitors. Wood instantly transforms your pristine and perhaps too hygienic home front into a modernist's pastoral playground. Wooden objects painted vibrant colors also serve as a fine distraction from structural disasters. You'll read how wood can transform an outdoor space, like a boring metal fence, into a spot with a homey and sweet atmosphere in Chapter 4.

Keep your eyes peeled for great items in the categories below on walks through your neighborhood or on special days (like bulk trash pickup in fancy neighborhoods):

- **Windowpanes** are jackpot finds. They make great room dividers—either hung from the ceiling (if your ceiling will support it) or by using their hinges and affixing them directly to a wall. I've used a particularly rustic square frame in place of a vanity mirror above my dresser. If the glass is not intact or if you're looking to make the frame lighter

Word to the Wise

Be sure to break glass out of old multipaned windows over a tarp or thick paper roll so you can easily (and safely) collect shards. Place glass shards in a sturdy cardboard box and seal before dumping them into the trash bin to keep broken glass from injuring yourself or sanitation workers.

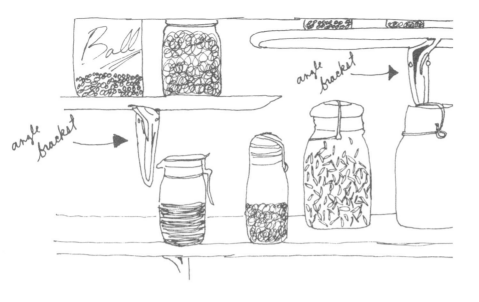

for hanging, you can carefully break out the remaining glass.

- I make a point of stalking **picture frames** of all sizes and shapes wherever I go. Setting something simple and elegant—like a glass bottle sporting a dried flower or two—in front of an open-back picture frame is a cheap and unique way to add character to your home.

- **Wood scraps** that sashay from one brightly painted color to the next, or anything wooden that looks like it washed in with the tide. After a quick trip to the hardware store, cool scraps can be made into an array of interesting and handy things, like coat racks or key holders. Major projects (involving saws and people who know how to operate them safely) can also leave you with room dividers, tabletops, and other marvels of modern carpentry.

- Abandoned **cabinet or full-sized doors** are fab finds for two reasons. One is the scavenged handle or drawer pull opportunity. I found a chic turquoise door handle on a ratty seventy-year-old door when neighbors on my block made renovations. Another cool thing to do with cabinet doors is to spruce them up with a layer of paint or a two-color scheme and use them as a cover for an unsightly view—a blank corner of a room, the backside of a room divider, or the lid of a storage unit.

- **Old shop shelves** (sturdy pieces of wood with angle brackets screwed to one side) make a great out-of-the-way entryway table for keys and curios. Use salvaged fence posts or other cool pieces of scavenged wood to create your own unique shelving.
- **Tables, chairs, and other furniture pieces** (more advanced finds). We picked up a vintage wooden dresser with gorgeous ornate engraving, totally free.

I once moved across the country with seven old windowpanes and a stack of orange fence posts that achieved higher priority in our tight minivan moving situation than the blender, measuring cups, stereo speakers, and my slightly functional art desk. That mass-produced stuff is replaceable; the found stuff is one of a kind.

Don't get me wrong, not every roadside relic is going to work in your house. Some of these items may, in fact, just be trash. The key is differentiating diamond-in-the-rough status from irreparably rough. And, of course, you have to have the carrying capacity (arms or wheels) to get the prize home.

Avoid wooden objects that display any of the following features:

- **Rotting or disintegrating planks.** A good piece of wood should be able to hold a nail without splintering off and breaking in two.

- **Something that needs a ton of work** (that you don't know how to do yourself). This will inevitably stress you out.
- **Particleboard.** It was awful when they bought it new, and it's even worse used. Just walk on by that wood-like composite.

make your house work for you

Working with what you already have is every thrifty house maven's secret weapon. Add the following special touches to upgrade what's already working. And feel free to forget the structural stuff, the home project headache, for the time being.

flowers

It's nice to have fresh flowers in the house, but when you're choosing between groceries and tulips, the decision is a no-brainer. Compromise and buy fresh flowers on days you're not restocking TP and laundry detergent. Specifically look for ones that dry prettily and keep their color. Jagged or ridged flowers keep their color in drying, whereas flowers with thin petals, like roses or gerbera daisies, for example, are more likely to turn brown or fall off as they dry. You

hip trick

Use a few non-matching vintage picture frames to display pretty paper, such as gift wrap, wallpaper samples, old maps, pages from magazines (*National Geographic*, *Arizona Highways*, and *Texas Highways* are some of my favorites), or illustrations from antique-y or fashionable calendars. Tie the quirkiness of the different frames together by painting them the same color, like white, a shocking red, or some other color that connects to your décor. Not only will it make that section of your wall pop, but paint will hide any chips or scratches in the old frames.

will want to hang the flowers upside down so they dry straight. My favorites for long-term display are generally members of the amaranth family, the most common being the globe amaranth flower. Deemed the "never-fading flower," these are of Brazilian origin, and come in lots of different colors—violet, red, yellow, white, and pink.

Other kinds of long-lasting flowers to look for:

- Cockscomb
- Mealy blue sage or lavender
- Statice

Special-occasion flowers (not great at drying well):

- Freesia makes a perfect pick-me-up. It smells divine, and its stems fit nicely in skinny bottle top openings, two or three to a bottle. You can spread a single bouquet around the house for fragrance all over.
- Tulips. Everyone loves tulips; Michael Pollan has an entire section about them in his book *The Botany of Desire*.
- Hydrangeas are pure luxury. They get droopy after a while, but we all need something fancy every now and then.

Flowers not only add color and texture to your room, but also, and perhaps more important, provide the opportunity to showcase your vase taste.

cover your vases

- Look for **vintage glass bottles** when you go to flea markets, estate sales, or thrift shops. They make excellent vases for spreading small portions of a bouquet around the house.

- Save your **small glass bottles**—like San Pellegrino's Aranciata bottles—or buy a couple of Mexican Cokes (a real delicacy in the United States because they're made with plain ol' sugar instead of high-fructose corn syrup) and save these taller-than-usual glass bottles. Skinny, small-mouth bottles make great vases for flashy single flowers.
- Use **mason jars** (pint- or quart-sized) for displaying full bouquets. You'll likely need to trim the stems so the vase doesn't tip over, though.

contain your joy

When you've left your flowers out on the table for too long (that is, you forgot to hang them upside down so they dry straight) you can clip the dried, droopy blooms and display them. Try displaying blooms (or other small curios) in any of these:

- Cute-shaped tart tins (they look like cookie cutters with bottoms)
- Ornate tea saucers or tiny plates from the thrift store
- Lids and rims of mason jars
- Small mason jars (if you have a lot of blooms, or if you have other objects—bottle caps, wine bottle corks, or matches—to add)

This brings me to a structural point, which must be addressed: you should have a place for everything. It's really okay to have a junk drawer. Some things just belong there: rubber bands, birthday candles, clothespins (the ones that aren't holding the rest of your house together), small things that you don't want to throw out.

bookish behavior

Always snatch up simple, sturdy bookcases when you see them roadside, at garage sales or antiques shops, or on Craigslist. Bookcases are the things people keep forever (or until they can afford built-ins), so never let a good one go to waste. Don't worry about scratches or wear. I carried a roadside find three-shelver home on the subway. My arm hurt for a week, but that bookcase is now absolutely indispensable.

In theory, I love the idea of color-coding or arranging books by jacket aesthetics. In practice, I'd never do it, at least not until I have an assistant who can find the one book I'm looking for at any given moment and a high-ceilinged library with floor-to-ceiling bookshelves and a sliding ladder to stash all the books that didn't make the "cute" cut.

Stick with color coding in your closet, arts and crafts bin, and underwear drawer, but on the bookshelf it's just not practical. You can spice up your bookshelves by arranging sections of books horizontally to break up the vertical monotony. If you have more room to work with, segregate smaller sections of books, like your poetry or picture books, from your fiction collection with knick-knacks and plants.

It's a good idea to go through your books once a year to thin the herd. (Moving apartments is a

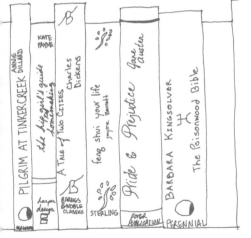

getting the most out of your home office space

- Take a shower in the morning, just as if you're going to work with other people.

- Get dressed, and not just in fresh pajamas.

- Adorn appropriately. The *Minimalista* blogger told me that she keeps her polish pretty and decks her fingers out with a sparkly ring or other bling to shake things up. Feeling excited about work can be nearly impossible when you're in your pajamas all day staring at your chipping manicure.

- Have on hand beverages or other rewards for productivity. (Margaritas are probably not the best idea in this case).

- Take breaks that involve water. Get the flow moving in your brain by doing a few dishes (not mopping the kitchen floor or cleaning the bathroom—that's just procrastination).

surefire book disposal mechanism.) Put the books you're not going to reread, or ones you're never going to read, on the stoop or curbside in a box with a sign marked "Free Books." Or better yet, donate them! It's good karma, and it keeps what's on your shelves current.

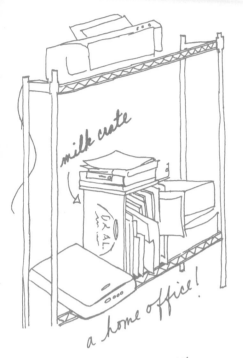

milk crate

a home office!

working from home, in the living room

Carving out space in your living room to work might be yet another thing you'll need to do with your 400-square-foot apartment. The work world is becoming more portable, more flexible with working situations—so it's likely that you, dear reader, are not working out of an office 100 percent of the time. If you must use your living room as a work space, here are questions to ask yourself to maximize the space (and your productivity).

setting yourself up for success, or where to put the desk

1. **Computing.** Does a network cable restrict you, or are you wireless?
2. **Phone location/cell reception.** Will you need to talk on the phone while you're at your computer? If so, it's best to position these elements near each other from the get-go.
3. **Lighting.** Are windows and natural light important to you? Do you need to be near a lamp?

getting down to business

1. **How well do you manage distractions** (kids, housework, Internet surfing) and how can you keep yourself on track? Setting little goals—like I did with finishing this section of the chapter—helps me achieve minor

successes and thus motivates me to stay focused, at
least for a little while longer.

2. **When should you give yourself a break?** Remember,
the home office is less prone to water cooler chat breaks,
unless you habitually talk to yourself. Home workers
commonly are more productive at home, so working for
four or five solid hours can actually be equivalent to an
eight-hour day at the office (shocker).

Now that we have the all-important living portions of your
home covered, we'll move on to areas in your home that are typi-
cally less viewed (by guests), but no less used (by you). The most
important way to gauge homifying success in your living areas
is to see if you feel comfortable just hanging out in them. Sometimes it takes a couple rearrangings to get things just right.

resources

Home project and style inspiration (people who can continue to
help you with the details):

- *Apartment Therapy* (book and blog).
- *The Nest: Home Design Handbook.*
- *Domino: Book of Decorating* or old *Domino* mags (out of
print now).
- Copies of *Red*, a British mag.
- Design Sponge blog.

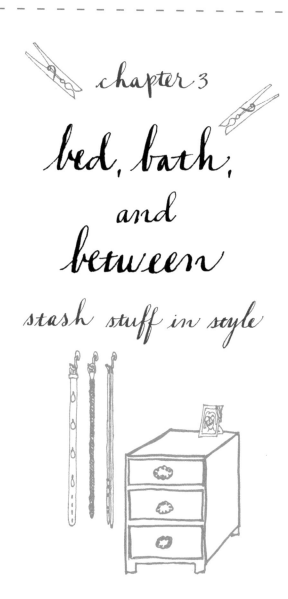

chapter 3

bed, bath, and between

stash stuff in style

Count this chapter as the "everywhere else" section for your room-by-room home-ifying adventure. Whether you've got a guest room or just a single room of your own, this chapter addresses utilizing and sprucing up your non-entertaining spaces. These are areas we use every day but perhaps give less thought or attention to.

I'm a total pack rat with borderline hoarder tendencies, and I always have more stuff than space. This chapter is a guide to striking a balance between packing all your tchotchkes away and having them crowd you out of your own house. As we head into the bathroom, the smallest and funkiest (in the uncool way) room of many houses, you'll notice distract-and-delight tactics paired with practical space-maximizing tips. Almost all dilemmas in these areas can be solved with a milk crate.

There are a zillion ways to be creative and make useful, cute solutions out of things you already have (or can find easily and cheaply), so take my suggestions as a way to get the brain ball rolling. Everyone's situation and circumstances are different, so try looking at your needs with an I-can-figure-this-out perspective, as opposed to an automatic gotta-run-to-Target-to-buy-more-plastic approach.

your library, leading a double life

Low on walls to divide your rooms? Consider a book partition for carving out a modicum of separation within your studio apartment or just adding depth to a room (and figuring out what the hell to do with the bookcase). Prettify the backside of a partitioning bookcase by draping a gauzy, simple cloth over it so that when you're in your new "room" you're not staring at an unsightly bookcase back. Or for a shorter bookcase, prop tall pieces of artwork or cool vintage cabinet doors against it.

I like shelving that's open on both sides for partitioning, like cube shelves, especially those reminiscent of Tetris pieces. This basic style is available in many different materials covering several price points, and goes nicely with most décor themes.

If your ceiling or wall permits, old windowpanes (the kind you'll purchase used or may find on the side of the road) make great partition tools. They're less about figuring out what to do with all your books, of course, and more about creating the illusion of separation, but they still make for fine space definers. You can also make your own multi-use partition out of things from the hardware store.

cinder block chic

My best friend and her hubby built a bookcase for me for my birthday one year. I'd just moved into a cool old duplex with a roommate, and my half of our situation was a single open room.

I needed a long, skinny wall-like object. Turns out four sturdy wood planks—two-by-eights, to be exact—and eight cinder blocks were the answer to my dilemma. Nathan, a punk rocker who's also pretty handy, knew exactly how to situate the cinder block bases (some vertical, most horizontal) and how high to safely build the structure, while Cassie, who remains a major source of my home décor inspiration, suggested a coat of lime green paint on the cinder blocks to spruce up the fact that I had punk rock shelving.

I stacked books along the lowest level of

Word to the Wise
Don't paint your cinder blocks on a rainy, humid weekend, like Nathan and Cassie did. You'll pull out your hair because the blocks won't dry for at least a week.

the upside of
an up cycle

When I moved to a new place
(with built-in bookcases,
hallelujah!), I used a plank
from my old bookshelves to
make a raised garden bed
frame, and I lined an unruly
outdoor area with my sassy
green cinder blocks, planting
succulents right inside
them. Learn other ways of
repurposing your stuff for
life in the great outdoors in
Chapter 4.

my homemade shelf to keep up safety measures
(that is, heavy stuff on the bottom) and stashed
CDs, photos, and even my stereo atop my custom
bookcase. Holes in the cinder blocks made for
cute knickknack displays.

bedroom décor

Set up your room based on the position of the
bed. Sometimes you only have one option due to
size constraints, the shape of your room, or the
position of its windows. I like to position my bed
so when I lie in it, my feet are pointing away from
the door.

Fancy bed frames are fun, but not exactly
affordable or realistic for everyone. The upside
to the basic metal bed frame is under-bed storage. Don't spend a bunch of money on a special
storage-drawer bed frame; just buy a few flat
tubs and a cool dust ruffle. You can always find
one of these basic frames on Craigslist, sometimes for $5 or $10.

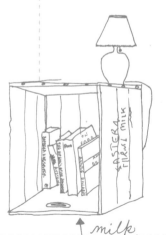

milk
crate

another bedside attraction

Use a sturdy vintage or contemporary milk crate for a
nightstand—just turn it on its
side, with the container part
facing out to form a little compartment to stash your journal

and bedside novel. If you are using a plastic milk crate that you don't love, drape it with a cute piece of fabric, wide enough to cover the top surface area and long enough to cover exposed sides.

Floating shelves are a great way for getting the official stuff— small lamps, clock, photographs of your pets, etc.—out of the way. A floating shelf hides the hardware involved in hanging it behind or actually inside the shelf where it meets the wall. They are available in most big-box stores and other home décor retail outlets. Just be sure to get one that will support the weight of what you have in mind to stash on it; weight limits will be listed on the installation instructions.

jewels jealousy

Three cute ways to show off jewelry in an accessible, no-dresser-surface-needed fashion:

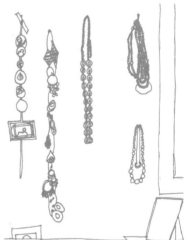

1. Hang pairs of earrings on a pretty ribbon pinned to the wall.
2. Find a fancy picture frame that works with your décor and affix a corkboard sheet to the back (or insert the sheet if there's an actual back to the frame). If you want something a little fancier, wrap the corkboard insert in a simple-patterned vintage cloth. You don't want some-thing too wild or you won't be able to find your jewelry in the pattern.
3. Peg those pretties right to the wall. Your necklaces fend for themselves in attractiveness; all you have to do is place a few of them on some sort of peg or nail

55

for display. Do two or three pegs depending on how many necklaces you own. Group similar-length strands together and arrange pegs in a staggered or stacked fashion. Fancy up the peg by using cute hooks in place of plain old nails.

bed linens

Plain white bed linens are an invitation for disaster. They may look fresh, light, and modern, but c'mon, for the reality of everyday use? Washing your comforter is sort of a pain in the ass.

Have at least two full sets of sheets, one for use most of the time and one for buying time between launderings (so you don't have to make up the bed after a long afternoon at the launderette). Have a third set if you receive houseguests often. Shop around for sale or end-of-season closeout options from places that sell organic, top-quality bed linens; Gaiam always has a good clearance section.

When buying sheets, think like you do with swimwear: yes, you can always go the route of a matching set, but more often than not mix-and-match sheets are a quirky, stylish, and definitely more affordable option (since single sheets are usually on clearance). Look for solid colors that complement each other and throw in a single pattern if it suits you.

Word to the Wise

Don't skimp on sheets; you and your bed are worth the investment. You won't consider the $40 price differential a positive after your subpar sheets fall apart and you need new ones, or when they become excessively scratchy instead of soft and sleep-worthy.

nifty ideas for bedroom accents

- Dress up your solid bed linens with a cool patterned throw pillow (or vice versa—accentuate your pretty patterned linens with a couple of solid-colored throw pillows).
- Dust ruffles are a great place to add some color or style to your room (and keep under-bed storage under wraps).
- Project: make your own throw pillow covers (even *I* could and did—and this as a pre–Hip Girl anti-seamstress).
- If you're averse to needle and thread, hit up the vintage circuit for cute pillows, linens orphaned from larger sets, and discarded curtains.
- Use a strip of vintage or cute fabric to tie back plain white or solid-colored curtains.
- Use interesting or bold-colored fabric to cover a couple of cheap stretched canvases (purchased from any arts and crafts store). Blocks of color make good use of an artless wall.

why organic?

Conventionally grown cotton is grown using toxic insecticides, herbicides, and/or fungicides, which pose health risks to people who live near the crops. Beyond human health, conventional cotton production compromises soil health and biodiversity, requiring ⅓ pound of chemical fertilizers to produce just 1 pound of cotton (about as much as is needed for one T-shirt). No thanks to all that.

ditch the horizontal prison

I hate miniblinds (except for wooden ones). I think the years I spent dusting our household, which was full of slatted metal, has something to do with my disdain. You can easily take these eighties décor relics down in rented apartments and put up cute and simple curtains in their place. Just stash the blinds with the hanging hardware and don't fill the holes, so reinstallation (when you move out or know your landlord's coming over) will be a snap.

window to your soul

There are three basic modes of treating your windows:

- Shades (pull-down or roll-up)
- Curtains (lighter-weight, breezy fabric accents)
- Drapes (heavy-duty statements and light blockage)

When it comes to selecting which ones are right for you, first figure out your window goals. Are you hoping for:

- Blocking heat caused by too much light (I wish this were my problem) → Shades or drapes
- Letting in light but blocking out the ability to see into your house from outside → Shades or curtains
- Blocking bright streetlights or the break of dawn while you slumber → Shades or drapes

shades

I ripped down the flimsy cloth accordion shades installed in our apartment at the start of our tenancy. These types of throw-away shades are bunk; you can't wash them (since they adhere directly to the window frame) and in our case there was no way to keep the shades up (except, thank goodness, for clothespins). Not all accordion shades are the cheap ones we had, but landlords often cut corners in rental properties.

If you go the shade route, I love the rice paper, bamboo, and other sheer and easily opened ones. Special shades also exist for the purpose of filtering out heat yet allowing light in.

In place of the cheapie accordion shades, I installed a Deka curtain wire from IKEA (which I will describe for you in full detail) and clipped a perfectly sized white tablecloth to the wire for a slideable, fancy-looking improvisation. You couldn't tell at all that we were using table linens to cover our main window.

A few months later I got around to borrowing a friend's sewing machine and making the curtains of our dreams (which, at their simplest, are just a rectangle or square shape with or without a wide hem to fit around a rod or clip to the Deka wire). The tablecloth was an excellent stand-in until I had the time to address the situation more creatively.

curtains

I'm not a flashy curtain rod person, but budget curtain rods are consistently ugly. My motto: make statements elsewhere. Valances can go to hell. They're like the monogrammed guest hand towel of the curtain world—not useful and, if done inexpertly, borderline Grandma's house (in the wrong sort of way).

This is one of the only times

Hip Trick

Need a quick curtain to cover an open shelf or unsightly utility area? Slice a cute thrift store pillowcase (with a wide hem at the open end) around the three sewn edges to open it up. Voilà—you have a pillowcase curtain ready to hang. Consult Chapter 6 for tips on finishing the edges when you have time.

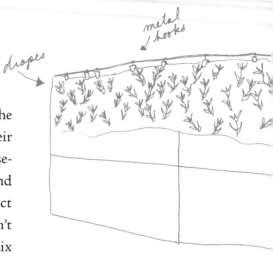

where I actually recommend schlepping your ass to IKEA and following the herd-ish maze straight to their curtain and window panel selections. Do not pass go, and stay focused or you'll collect two hundred things you don't need that will fall apart in six months.

deka wire

IKEA's Deka curtain wire setup is superbly useful, simply designed, and even reusable (if you move, take it with you to reinstall again). For $4.99, you're in business covering window spans of up to 118 inches. The best part of this construction is that the little clips are fashioned sort of like a clothesline and allow you to affix fabric to the window as a curtain without needing to sew anything (unless you're finishing edges). Need I say more?

Well, yes: you have to actually, physically go into an IKEA store to buy the Deka wire. You can't currently order it online. Insane? Yes. Buy a handful, like I did, and save yourself a trip in the future. There's also a version that fits around the exterior of the window frame, as opposed to this setup, where the wire sits within the window frame. Choose either version to suit your specific window needs.

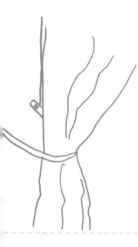

If you get (or make) curtains that are just fabric folded over itself to form the rod pocket (not fancier tabs that actually show the curtain rod), you can get away with the simple tension rod, my other all-time curtain-hanging favorite.

drapes

Many curtain ideas apply to drapes, but beware that rods may need to be a bit sturdier to support heavy fabrics. Also keep in mind that blackout fabric can be affixed to an existing drape to make the room darker, if needed.

Thrift store drapes are a great option. Especially since IKEA hit everyone's radar, I've seen plenty of great-condition IKEA options at thrift stores. You'll find them for a fraction of the price and relatively unblemished (because drapes are a really hard thing to stain). Most drape hooks—the things that hold heavier drapes back, anchoring them to each side of the window—on the market are ugly. I ended up picking up two ridiculously cheap plant hooks (I found them much cheaper than drape hooks!) and affixing them to the wall to hold back our thick red velvet drapes in the daytime.

You're going to need a drill for heavy-duty window treatment installations. Read up on getting tight with your tool kit in Chapter 7. Many of the simpler setups can be installed with a hammer, a screwdriver, and a ruler.

bathroom décor

My current apartment has a pedestal sink that doesn't attach to the wall properly, and no shelving beyond a wood-framed medicine cabinet (an interesting décor choice in the context of a black-and-white-tiled 1950s-style motif). This is my flawed palette, and I'm not really worried about it. My real friends will not judge me.

Word to the Wise

Don't undertake curtain rod installation after a long day of moving and unpacking. It's a bright-eyed, bushy-tailed kind of job that demands patience and careful attention, or you'll end up with cockeyed curtain rods.

The bathroom is the smallest room in the house; therefore, this is not the place to make bold statements. Your bathroom should conjure clean, light feelings, or at least not gross people out. Keep it clean, literally and decoratively.

paint job blues

If you only paint one area of your home, then I suggest painting the bathroom. Nothing about painting is as quick and easy as design and décor sites assert, but there are ways to be smart about it.

Once upon a time, I lived in an apartment that an obviously color-blind person (or manic color-coder) occupied before me. The bathroom walls were all different colors: deep plum over the shower, a two-tone pink and baby blue surrounding the toilet, and a single shade of pink on the wall behind the medicine cabinet and sink. Clearly, this bathroom needed a paint makeover (which I finally managed to undertake a full year after moving in).

If you're in a similar predicament or just looking to make your place a bit nicer than what the landlord is lending you, consider "oops" paint—paint that retailers or hardware stores custom-mixed but either the customer who ordered it didn't pick it up or the color did not turn out to the customer's liking. It's a good option for budget-conscious folks who aren't super-attached to one specific color. When I buy a house and need to paint every wall in the house, I fully intend to buy a 100 percent milk-based, solvent-free, or less-toxic alternative (for both me and the planet), but for now, I'm opting to paint smaller spaces and single walls to accentuate my rented walls. So "oops" paint will do!

Things to look for and keep in mind when selecting paint:

62

- Choose one with no or low VOCs—volatile organic compounds. That's the stuff that vaporizes over time and climbs into your lungs when you breathe.
- If you don't see anything about VOCs listed, try to steer clear of products with ingredients like formaldehyde, ammonia, acetone, and odor masking agents.
- Consider opacity or hide—how many coats will it take to achieve the color promised by the cute little paint chip.
- Mind if you will need to prime the surface (apply a special coat of base paint, usually white or gray) before applying color; some paints are self-priming, so you use less paint (and energy) when all is said and done.

don't be shelfless

I have a real knack for renting places with shelfless bathrooms. If I'm lucky, I'll get either a medicine cabinet or a below-sink cabinet, but usually not both.

I solved my shelflessness (and linen closet deficiency) with a milk crate shelf for towels in my newly painted yellow bathroom. This type of shelf can be tricky in super-tight quarters since you'll need to hang it high enough so you don't hit your head or run into it coming in and out of the room. Affixing a milk crate to the wall is simple. Use long screws with a wide enough head to catch the grid (so it doesn't slide right off the wall). A longer-bodied screw hook would work perfectly here; see Chapter 7 for the lowdown on hardware.

Hip Trick

For the lowest-tech shelving enhancement ever, just place a milk crate or similar sturdy, cute bin on an existing large shelf. You'll add depth, structure, and additional storage surface to the bigger space.

63

Another quick fix for adding shelving to your miniature bathroom is an over-the-toilet shelf. These stand on long legs over the toilet tank and are hardly brag-worthy, but they're inexpensive and easy to find. A layer of low-VOC spray paint can transform the piece, at the very least, into a unique and quite possibly even charming or vintage-looking place to stash essential stuff. (Always apply spray paint outside, no matter how safe the manufacturer says it is to spray inside with ventilation; check out Chapter 5 to read up on why you want to keep your indoor air free of chemicals.)

shower curtains that don't suck

I've been through nearly every type of shower curtain you can buy in an attempt to save both the planet and my sanity. Vinyl sorta creeps me out, and I had a hell of a time with mildew on all the materials that say they won't mildew, including cotton, hemp, and even polyester.

Because of my bad luck, I now gravitate toward the polyester "hotel" shower curtain liner for its sheer innocuousness (and the upwardly mobile option to add a pretty outer curtain someday, when I can afford Marimekko). These liners are usually white or neutral hues and cost anywhere from $12 to $16. If you wash it regularly and curb mildew as soon as you see it, your liner will look nice for years to come.

Speaking of mildew prevention efforts . . . old apartments usually leave much to be desired in the ventilation department. Ours lacks vent fans in

Hip Trick

Install a water-saving showerhead. They start at just $15, cut your water usage by almost half, and increase the pressure of the water coming out (which makes showering oh so nice).

64

both the kitchen and bathroom (fancy that). If you're in a similar situation, or just want to cool off the stifling bathroom during summer months, pick up a small fan, either clamp-style or a small desktop type, to get some air flowing in your bathroom.

Be prepared, though. Even with officially administered ventilation, mildew happens. After about six months of use, I discovered spots near the bottom of our hotel-quality liner where it wasn't drying out fully. Some simple steps to avoid running into this problem and extend the life of your liner include:

- Stop buying vinyl shower curtains.
- Lug a fan into the bathroom and keep it there. I just replaced our 5-inch clip fan with a deluxe 13-inch fan. I'm serious about ventilation.
- Wring out your shower curtain or liner after you turn off the shower water.
- Place your all-cloth bathmat (rubber-bottomed mats are a mildew magnet in poorly ventilated bathrooms) over the edge of the tub. Gather your curtain or liner loosely behind the area where the cloth bathmat is covering the tub edge. Don't scrunch it up tightly, but spread it out over the length of your bathmat. This allows air into the shower stall from the sides and keeps the tub from incubating areas of mildew where it touches your liner/curtain. Pull it back down an hour later so guests don't see your crazy mildew prevention efforts.

Don't fret if you do notice mildew spots. It doesn't say horrible things about you. The shower curtain, like any of your household linens, still needs a wash every now and then. Read up on laundering in Chapter 6; you'll see it's not the pain you thought it was.

quick chic:
five bathroom décor dos and don'ts

DO:

1. Use small jars or cups to hold medicine cabinet supplies like Q-tips, nail care tools, makeup pencils, or cotton balls.
2. Decorate with neatly folded linens on a behind-the-toilet rack or any other type of bathroom shelving.
3. Stash a handful of magazines in an accessible location if you have a spare shelf.
4. Relocate occasionally used beauty supplies, tools, and bathroom goods to a nearby closet to free up space for everyday essentials. Contain the excess in individual tubs or cute bins (if it's an open shelf). Clementine boxes make great beauty-stuff stashers.
5. Attempt to hone a color scheme in your bathroom, which sometimes means catering to existing wall and floor tiles. Coordinate linen colors so they don't stand out amidst the context of your existing color scheme.

DON'T:

1. Hold on to makeup and skin care products that have long-past (or don't even have) expiration dates. It's good to use products that expire; don't buy the Twinkies of the body and face care product world, things that can sit indefinitely on the shelf due to additives and preservatives.

2. Place rolled-up towels in a basket on the floor unless you're a meticulous weekly cleaner. I don't know why the bathroom floor gets so gross so fast, but you'll be doing laundry way more than you bargained for by stacking clean towels down there.

3. Keep magazines in an unkempt pile on the floor. Disarray in small spaces sucks.
4. Cram all your bathroom goods or unwieldy toiletries onto your precious shelving.
5. Choose dark bath linens if you have a small bathroom. A surefire way to make a tiny bathroom even tinier is to load up on dark accents. We opted for a cream and tan towel scheme in our black and white (and wood) bathroom, with red accents infused sparingly so as not to close up the little space we do have.

grown-up towels

Now is the time to ditch those mismatched, fraying pre-college towels (or make dishrags out of them to not be wasteful). They've served you (and maybe your parents) well; now serve yourself well by picking out towels that make you feel warm and fuzzy.

On typical laundry dates, my laundering pal helps me fold as we wrap things up. (I inevitably have more, laundering for two and all.) One afternoon, as she finished folding miscellaneous towels, my laundry pal said, "Here are your rags." I snatched my bathroom hand towel and washcloths from the stack indignantly. Her not-surprising mistake got me thinking.

67

If you can't distinguish between the towels that dry your body and those you clean the bathroom with, something's wrong with this picture. Towels are a relatively easy way to fancy things up without spending half your rent money. Shoot for organic if you find sale ones (like online in Gaiam's clearance section), head to overstock stores like T. J. Maxx and Tuesday Morning, or trek out to manufacturers' outlet stores on your next road trip.

storage and the lack thereof

Closet space multiple choice: So, you're not going to the Container Store and buying an all-customized closet organization system because:

    a. You're renting
    b. You're broke
    c. Your closet walls are drywall and can barely hold a nail
    d. You don't have a closet

If any of the above apply to you, it's time to proceed to closet plan B.

Under-bed space is a perfect place to stash bulky or seasonal items like linens, sweaters, swimsuits, or even gift wrap accoutrements.

Stash seasonal clothes or shoes in large Rubbermaid tubs in a coat closet. They're stackable and offer a raised surface shelf for other items. Using all available space is essential when you haven't much of it in the first place.

accessories

The beloved milk crate saves the day once again. Use a plastic milk crate (or some other sort of see-through-ish box) to stash purses, hats, and other occasional-use items. Alternatively, hang a long piece of twine from the closet bar (or nail it to the wall) and clothespin baseball caps, hats, and other light accessories to the twine.

Hang traditionally designed belts from a standard hanger by looping the belt buckle through the hanger's hook. For your more fashionable belts, just hook the belt together as it's worn but through the hanger.

I prefer back-of-the-door shoe organizers to ones that take up valuable space on your closet hanging bar. If for some reason you have actual shelving in your actual closet, stacking shoe boxes with Sharpie-detailed descriptions of the footwear contents is a good method for getting seasonal shoes off your closet floor. Don't waste your Polaroid film on snapshots of your shoes; if you have so many shoes that a few written words won't jog your memory of the contents, then a major shoe cleanout is in order.

linens

I've spent many years, in many linen-closet-less apartments, figuring out what to do with spare sheets, guest bedding, and towels that don't fit in the bathroom, or anywhere nearby.

Hip Trick

Most standard metal bed frames will need the wheels attached in order to accommodate the height of storage tubs. If you don't have the kind with wheels, find a set of bed frame feet for $10 to elevate the frame or return to your roots with the handy dorm trick of stacking your bed frame on cinder blocks for added storage space. An extra long dust ruffle will hide the whole affair beautifully.

how to fold a fitted sheet without going insane

Follow these six easy steps for smoothing out your (faux) linen closet or just impressing friends at the launderette. The big fitted sheet secret: it's all about corners, people; make a square out of what really isn't and then just make it smaller.

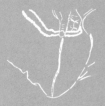

STEP 1: Locate any two corners that are next to each other, and stick your index fingers into their tips (where the corners of your bed would go).

STEP 2: Bring your index fingers together and peel one corner down on top of the other. You should have both corners resting on one fingertip. Set this end down and repeat for the other set of corners.

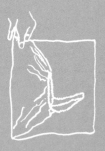

STEP 3: Bring your two sets of corners together, peeling one set over the other in the same fashion as Step 2.Your sheet is now folded in quarters with all four of the rounded corners stacked neatly in one tip.

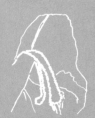

STEP 4: This is the point where most people start getting frustrated. Lay sheet down carefully on bed or folding table and do your best to make the quartered sheet into a square shape. Do this by folding the flaps of the two edges with the rounded corners into an L-shape.

STEP 5: Take a deep breath and fold your new square-shaped sheet over three times to make a long skinny rectangle.

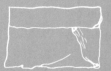

The corner where the L-shape meets might give you trouble in this step. Manage inner lumpiness by ensuring that the crux of the L doesn't get bunched up as you fold. You can stick your hand in and smooth it out after you fold the first portion down if that's easier.

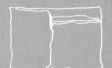

STEP 6: Make it smaller again. Hint: don't force three even folds here; your sheet will be wider on one end than the other, so think of it like a puzzle and play around with it.

Press, crease, and voilà! Appreciate a job well done!

Right now we're blessed with an inordinately large pantry closet, which has effectively morphed into our pantry/linen/medicine/mailing-supplies closet.

As chaotic as this sounds, each shelf is organized and contained. Linens are folded neatly (so they actually fit), medicines and bathroom supply excesses are in separate containers (and accessibly convenient to pull down and dig through), food is sequestered to a single shelf, and a space-saver shelf utilizes space between shelves for food storage items like cling wrap, parchment paper, and waxed paper sandwich bags.

Stick linens in a plastic tub or two (with lids) when you must store them in the highest or lowest spots in your closet, to keep them clean and dust-free.

putting it all together

You've done it! You made it through the homey home basics section using things you found, bought on the cheap, or just improvised. Move on to Part II, where we'll cover the (possibly daunting) acts of domesticity that involve caring for your décor and home goods. Don't forget to throw yourself (and your house) a party; rewards are the most important part of homekeeping.

I'll leave you with a few quick décor tips as a Part I recap.

five décor dos and don'ts

DO:

1. Use rugs to distract visitors from crappy linoleum. Textured or colorful rugs are perfect distract and delight components.

2. Localize lighting in your living room. Table lamps and hanging lamps are great ways to add flair to your house. My living room lighting centerpiece is a standard compact fluorescent bulb hanging inside an antique wire birdcage.

3. Throw a piece of heavyweight fabric over that ugly couch you bought at the thrift store. It's an inexpensive and classy fill-in until you have enough money to re-upholster it as intended.

4. Stack large coffee table books alongside of a couch or chair to create a makeshift table.

5. Use a mirror in the place of art to make the space look larger.

DON'T:

1. Buy an area rug that will be a pain in the ass to clean (especially if you have pets or kids). Like you really need a $100 dry cleaning bill every few months. Key words: machine washable.

2. String Christmas lights around the ceiling perimeter. You're no longer in your college dorm room. Try winding a strand into a tight ball and hanging it like a lamp. Extra points for getting an LED strand, which will last longer and use less energy than the standard bulb strands.

3. Hang a tapestry on your wall (unless you live in a yoga studio or acupuncture office).

4. Stack more than two or three books on your bedside stand or coffee table; they just take up useful space and say "I need a bookshelf," not "Look at my great taste in books."

5. Position a mirror directly opposite a window; it's bad feng shui juju. Plus you don't want to reflect all the light brought in from the outdoors right back out of the room.

resources

books

Peruse your bookstore! You'll find tons of books on feng shui, painting, and organizing things to fit your individual decorating needs.

web

» remodelista.com
  Great ideas for sprucing up areas of the house with DIY and low-cost solutions.

» theimprovisedlife.com
  Lots of creative improvisation to be had here.

Part II

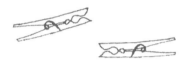

Impressive Acts
of Domesticity:
Do Try This at Home

chapter 4

outdoor spaces

make nice with
the great outdoors

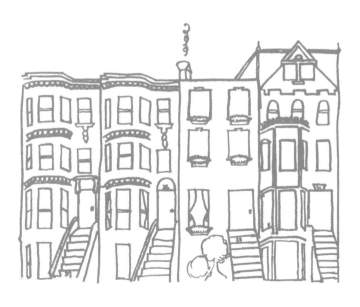

As this chapter quickly exploded well beyond my allotted word count, I soon realized that a short overview of gardening is impossible. There are entire books out there devoted exclusively to soil, compost, container gardening, spotted bugs, removing dirt from your fingernails, etc.

Gardening is one of those areas where you can easily suffer from TMI (too much information). It's actually better to jump right in with a few basics under your belt and save reading the countless books, magazines, and online tips for when you encounter specific issues. The problem with too much book smarts in the beginning is the absence of reality, that is, what's really going to happen when you try it yourself. No one can tell you that; no one's variables are exactly like yours.

Here's what Michael Pollan has to say about all this (from an interview in *Organic Gardening* magazine): "We read books to learn how to garden; then the reality turns out to be more complicated. It doesn't come out the way it's supposed to in the book, and there are always surprises." As you're probably well aware, he also wrote a whole book—*The Botany of Desire*—on how humans have attempted to control our ecosystems with varying levels of success.

I'm not a master gardener; I have successfully planted, tended, and consumed my own vegetables and herbs. There have been plenty of surprises, sure, but that's the most intriguing part of it all. The garden is a study in slowness, patience, the everyday. If any of these things eludes you, don't fret; just start small.

As with everything in this book, there are many levels of involvement (and means/capacities). Just because you don't have actual outdoor space doesn't mean you should pitch the idea of gardening out the window. Instead, stick with the window and establish a sunny ledge as your home's food production region.

Or consider gardening on your rooftop. What you learn from tending a few pots will lend itself to future plans of extending into the ground or just growing more and working smarter next year.

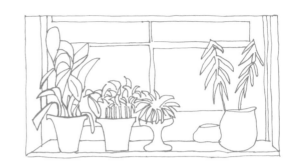

So what does all this mean to you, beginning gardener? It means freedom. Freedom to mess up, freedom to discover and incorporate slowness into your life. One single basil plant will shift you, no matter how slightly, toward freedom from the industrial food chain and large companies dictating what you put in your mouth.

Before we head to the great outdoors, let's check out (or reinstate) green space inside your home. After all, not everyone gets to stake a claim to their own patch of exterior nature.

frantic foliage

I have a notoriously bad relationship with houseplants. The great indoors and I came to terms a few years ago when I managed to grow a new devil's ivy plant from a cutting of a larger plant. After living in a plastic cup for about eight months, this tenacious variety sprouted roots, at which point I relocated it into soil. After this migration my plant carried on a static existence for the next year, not growing, but staying alive (which I count as success). One house move and a west-facing window later, my plant took off, climbing the walls and shooting limbs in every direction. The indoor plant gospel rang from my kitchen window: places where plants look good are not always places where the sun shines.

Up to this point, I never gave interior conditions much

79

thought. My plant planning consisted of weekend mornings spent strolling through aisles of pretty plants of all shapes and sizes at my local nursery. I selected things I liked and hoped for the best. I soon discovered that good intentions mean nothing when it comes to plants and their multiple, variable needs. Buying the wrong kinds of indoor plants is a long, fraught process of tearing up your money and throwing it in the compost pile.

snake plant

have your houseplant and keep it alive, too

There are a few considerations to keep in mind when choosing houseplants:

1. *Light.* How does light fade in and out of the proposed plant space? Where you think a houseplant should go and where a houseplant will get enough light to survive may not match up. Some of you are lucky enough to have too much light for certain plants (but for the record, most plants don't see this as a problem).

2. *Temperature, humidity, or other desired conditions.* Some plants need a greenhouse-y atmosphere, not your radiator-gone-wild, 500-degrees-in-the-winter apartment. Don't buy these varieties. Ask the people at the plant nursery before you buy anything. Or better yet, get a copy of *Taylor's Guide to Houseplants* if you're doing most of your leafy tinkering indoors.

cast iron plant

I'm used to barely maintaining plant life in my cave-like, low-light apartment situation, a challenge to houseplant survival. But I have hopes of moving somewhere one day where my windows won't face north.

spotted evergreen

Six houseplants that won't die in your cave (i.e., low-light best bets):

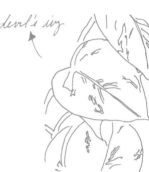

kangaroo vine

devil's ivy

grape ivy

1. Cast-iron plant (*Aspidistra elatior*).
   This member of the lily family tops my chart with a description in *Taylor's* of abilities to withstand "poor soil, low light and minimal care." This one also stole my heart by earning its nickname by surviving in dim, coal-fumed Victorian-era households. If they could keep this plant alive, then so can you.
2. Kangaroo vine (*Cissus antarctica*).
   Any plant with Antarctica in its scientific name must be able to survive in my house. This is a hanging plant, thus a great option for sprucing up small spaces.
3. Grape ivy (*Cissus rhombifolia*).
   A relative of the kangaroo vine, perhaps the most arty of the low-lighters with its faceted leaves.
4. Spotted evergreen (*Aglaonema costatum*).
   Looks sort of like a leopard print philodendron with big leaves.
5. Devil's ivy (*Epipremnum aureum*).
   You could not kill this plant if you tried.
6. Snake plant (*Sansevieria trifasciata*).
   This one has the double benefit of fitting in tight spaces (since it's tall and skinny) and filtering indoor air.

None of these are flashy, showy plants. In fact, they are the exact same plants you'll find at any fluorescent-lit office building or in shopping malls that don't have skylights.

81

did you know . . .

Houseplants improve indoor air quality by removing VOCs (discussed in Chapter 3) like formaldehyde and benzene and by absorbing carbon dioxide. The chemicals find their way to the plant's roots, where microbes do the work of breaking them down into energy or food.

quick chic: five indoor/outdoor décor dos and don'ts

DO:

1. Spruce up a plain ol' chain-link fence with old windowpanes or vintage wooden picture frames (ones you don't mind getting weather-worn).

2. Run a clothesline between any two sturdy things you can tie the line to directly or with screws (e.g., a fencepost, deck post, etc.). If you're strapped for outdoor space, buy an indoor line kit that winds back into the casing between uses.

3. Use simple hardware to hang a hammock somewhere in your yard or common area. This way it's easy to take down if you share the space with others. Pick up two 3-foot pieces of midweight chain and two screw links (like a carabiner that has a screw bolt), and you're in hammock-hanging business.

4. Utilize whatever space you have for growing plants, be it windowsills, a fire escape, a stoop, a roof, or even a small yard. Remember that hanging space might be one of your best assets. I've suspended my strawberry jar from the neighbor's deck, where it'll get enough sun to fruit all summer long.

5. Line a walkway with cinder blocks painted bright colors and plant succulents (or other inedible native plants) in the holes as a low-cost way to spruce up your front or back yard.

DON'T:

1. Place food plants directly underneath your decorative windowpane-lined fence or wall; little paint chips will drift down into the soil, and consuming hundred-year-old lead paint is not good for you.

2. Keep your clothespins on the line all the time because weather exposure will cause them to mildew and rust. Instead, stash them on a coat hanger in your closet and bring it outside with you when you hang your clothes or linens.

3. Hang your hammock somewhere you don't want to sit, like the corner of the yard that meets the corner where the neighbor's dog routinely poops. At the time it seemed like a perfectly good idea to string up my hammock underneath our upstairs neighbors' deck; then I realized that deck debris would fall on my face if anyone happened to be walking overhead.

4. Assume all windows are the same. I've killed more than my share of cute succulents by hoping my north-facing window would be sufficient for sun-guzzling foliage. Figure out your window's orientation and make decisions about plants from there.

5. Use painted cinder blocks or wood planks to make garden boxes for food plants. Painted things might leach toxins you don't want to consume into the soil.

Hip Trick

Dress up a sorta boring, low-light plant champ with a cool pot. Be sure your chic pot has drainage holes in it, though, if you don't want to be figuring out how to drill holes in ceramic on your day off.

introduction to container gardening

If you need inspiration to try growing something edible, consider the scary, invasive scope of the industrial food system; the nutritional benefits of consuming food that has not traveled for days on a semitruck; or doing your part to snatch up floating molecules of carbon dioxide via plant foliage.

Years of tinkering and observing what's going on in my pots has helped me put things in perspective, mainly allowing me to realize that I'm apparently not the center of the universe. It's funny what a few plants with their own ideas of fun can do for your outlook. I've managed to grow and eat my own vegetables and herbs for a few seasons now. I like it, and after you put aside fears of failure, you might like it too.

As you move through understanding the whys of the garden (and I don't think anyone ever gets all of them), you'll gain confidence and start to see things you've never noticed before, like the way lettuce slowly unfolds or how sprouts emerge from their seeds in a forward-bend-like position.

Don't read too much before you start, or you might not ever start. There are so many factors involved, most of them living (read: unpredictable) and at the microbial level. Leave complexity to your soil; basic gardening should be a learn-as-you-go thing, no expertise required to start. First rule of plant tending: relax!

potting a plant

This skill applies to both indoor plant tending and container gardening; the method is exactly the same. It's really all about drainage.

The essentials:

- ◆▸ Something with holes in the bottom
- ◆▸ Rocks or broken pieces of terra-cotta or dishware
- ◆▸ Organic potting mix
- ◆▸ Vermiculite or coir (optional)
- ◆▸ Fertilizer (for indoor plants) or compost (for outdoor plants)
- ◆▸ Topsoil or mulch (for outdoor plants)
- ◆▸ Bricks (optional)

1. Buy pots with drainage holes. Or if you're poking/drilling your own drainage holes in something like a food-grade 5-gallon bucket, don't be stingy. Look under existing pots (depending on the size you're working with) and use their drainage hole sizes and positionings as a guide.
2. Line the bottom of the pot with 1 to 2 inches of rocks or pot shards to allow extra room for drainage. Some books say you can use Styrofoam packing peanuts, but nowadays it's hard to tell which ones are true Styrofoam and which ones are planet-friendly, biodegradable doppelgangers. You don't want a pot bottom full of decomposing faux Styrofoam. Stick to broken stuff, or better yet, get a huge bag of landscaping/pond rocks for $5. (Don't buy decorative rocks; you're wasting your money.)
3. Though potting mix is designed specifically for containers, you can always add extra fluff to keep the soil from compacting. Vermiculite or coir (coconut husk fiber) are both good fluffing additives, but avoid peat moss since it's a nonrenewable resource. Never pack down soil in your pot.

85

4. When the pot is about half full of soil, I drop in a scoop of organic fertilizer to get the soil microbes and bacteria going, and for outdoor plants, I add a handful of compost. Follow directions on your fertilizer bag for proper proportions.

5. If the plant's root ball is tightly compacted, gently loosen the roots with your fingers, as if you're untangling a knot from long hair.

6. Fill pot with potting mix to 2 inches from the top of the pot, and add topsoil to top off the pot. Don't worry—when you water for the first time, the soil will settle, leaving an inch or so of space between the top of the pot and the soil. Topsoil (or mulch) protects and insulates your soil life, a good idea for plants that are exposed to full-sun (otherwise your plants will dry out faster and develop a brittle top layer).

7. Set larger pots (like 5-gallon buckets) on two or three bricks to assist drainage. You never want your pots to sit in a pool of water; the roots will rot.

8. Water thoroughly, until you see water coming out of the drainage holes.

I like how *Taylor's Guide to Houseplants* explains how to properly extract cuttings and propagate plants.

watering basics

How to water your plants:

- **Indoor plants.** Water sparingly. Let them dry out completely. Root rot (from overwatering) is the most common killer of indoor plants. Your plants will tell you when they're thirsty; they'll droop slightly. My low-light plants usually go weeks between waterings.

- ►► ***Outdoor plants.*** Water when dry, which usually means once daily. Hot, sunny summer days (combined with container scenarios) will suck the moisture right out of your plants. The best way to make sure your plants are getting enough water is to touch the soil. Poke your fingers down a few inches and feel around; if it's bone dry, then your plants are thirsty.

As you get fancier (I have yet to do this), you can buy or make a soaker hose for a slow-drip deep-watering setup. I like to use dark-colored glass bottles (like wine bottles or similarly sized ones) as inverted drip waterers in my container plants during especially hot times. The plants will take water as needed (like you do at the office water cooler), thanks to simple physics.

short course on fertilizer

Any bag of fertilizer you pick up will have three numbers written on it. Those numbers stand for the nitrogen, phosphorus, and potassium (N-P-K) ratios. Some fertilizers cater to certain types of plants or specific soil needs: a 4-6-4 ratio will be better for flowering parts of plants (vegetables included), and a 7-2-1 will help acidify overly alkaline soil with a nitrogen blast. I selected a fertilizer this year with mycorrhizal fungi to balance and assist microbial and bacterial growth.

Word to the Wise

Avoid watering outdoor plants during the day, even if your plants are wilted and thirsty. Direct sunlight heats up the soil, and the heated water could burn the roots of the plants. Instead, water in the morning or evening hours, and stick to spraying the soil, not the leaves.

Fill your watering can immediately after you empty it and let the water sit at room temperature until you use it again (twenty-four hours). Tap water can contain any number of chemicals, like chlorine, as remnants from the sanitization process, and these chemicals aren't great for plants, especially container plants. Leaving the water overnight allows smaller, volatile chemicals to dissipate into the air.

For beginning purposes, start with a basic, all-purpose fertilizer (something similar to an 8-2-4 ratio) at first and expand your knowledge as you go along, amending soils with both fertilizer and companion plants (beans are an excellent source of nitrogen for your soil). Avoid synthetic fertilizers—ones with really high numbers in the ratio—and instead stick with organic and natural choices, which are nonpolluting to the watershed and don't salinate the soil (make it too salty), which would kill beneficial microbes who are working to make your soil richer.

Alternate fertilizer feedings with applications of worm castings (which you can buy by the bag at any organic garden shop). Worm poop is balanced—equal in N-P-K ratios—and a perfect addition to any kind of soil.

my bucket garden

This year I planted my garden using six 5-gallon buckets from my local hardware store. You can also find these food-grade plastic buckets in restaurants, pickle and mayonnaise tubs in particular; ask around wherever you go. Do not use buckets that were once filled with plaster, paint, or any other nonfood item.

I drilled a bunch of holes in the bottoms of my buckets (which was oddly soothing, but more on that in Chapter 7), dropped some pond rocks in to assist drainage, filled them with a local potting soil mix, and voilà! Serious container gardening ensued. My six buckets are now planted with edibles:

- Raspberries
- Carrots
- Dutch wax beans
- Tomatoes

- Bell peppers
- Chioggia beets
- Double-yield cucumbers

Instead of bricks to elevate each bucket, I lined my buckets up along two parallel two-by-fours to create a little pedestal and air tunnel underneath them.

four times the charm

I've repotted my lone alpine strawberry plant several times. First I went from a 3-inch pot to a hanging basket; then I put it in a strawberry jar (a kind of pot that has holes in the sides to create more fruiting area). Then I learned that the alpine variety doesn't reproduce via runners like all the other strawberry plant varieties; I needed to put separate plants in each of the holes for a higher yield. So I severed two new shoots and their roots and planted them in the holes in the jar. (Hell, if a strawberry plant has to die for me to learn how to take a root cutting, then so be it. I'll buy another for $4 and be all the wiser for it.)

Then I couldn't resist buying an Ozark Beauty at the farmers' market. This one is an ever-bearing variety that spreads via runners. Bingo! All I needed to do was add it to one of the holes in my jar. Not so easy as envisioned, but my not-so-ideal planting situation has worked out just fine.

The moral of this tidbit: planting rules and guidelines are not set in stone; there's not just one way to do things. All plants involved are thriving (even the rogue cuttings).

89

guerrilla gardening

In addition to my container garden, spread out between my neighbor's back deck and our front stoop area, I also took over the little 3-foot-square concrete, dirt, and debris patch just outside our stoop. I moved my globe amaranth starts, a few native plant containers, and my most invasive stoop garden plant, mint, for a trial run in the wide world of Hancock Street. I'm considering moving my stoop beets container to this patch too, since it's a much better sun spot and since neighborhood kids and passersby haven't disturbed my plot since it debuted.

I built a three-sided frame around it using four 12-inch screws and a 2-foot section of fine mesh chicken wire cut into three strips. Reclaiming this space from debris and trash accumulation and seeing it generally unscathed for months renews my faith in humanity. I peek outside occasionally, watching for the occasional smile or nod of appreciation as people walk by.

what to grow?

Your very first task in plotting a garden of any sort should be to visit a local plant nursery to track down your local planting chart according to hardiness zone. This sublimely useful diagram shows what vegetables thrive in your ecological zone, what to start indoors or seed directly in the garden, and time frames for each.

First, find your hardiness zone by plugging in your zip code on the National Gardening Association's website: garden.org/zipzone. These charts

Word to the Wise

Community garden plots are a fine idea in theory, but unless gardening is your only hobby, you live next door to the garden, or you can work out watering shifts with other plot holders, you might instead consider a guerrilla patch on the sidewalk outside your house. You don't need the daily demands of the garden to raise your stress level.

are not always easy to track down, but they *do* exist. It's easier
once you know what you're looking for.

Here's my New York City/Zone 6 chart as an example:

NEW YORK CITY PLANTING CALENDAR

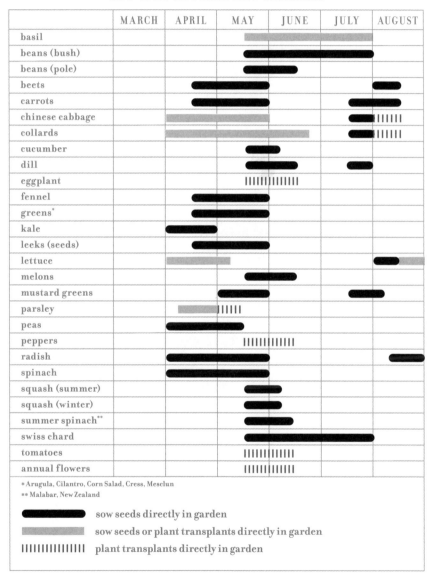

	MARCH	APRIL	MAY	JUNE	JULY	AUGUST
basil						
beans (bush)						
beans (pole)						
beets						
carrots						
chinese cabbage						
collards						
cucumber						
dill						
eggplant						
fennel						
greens*						
kale						
leeks (seeds)						
lettuce						
melons						
mustard greens						
parsley						
peas						
peppers						
radish						
spinach						
squash (summer)						
squash (winter)						
summer spinach**						
swiss chard						
tomatoes						
annual flowers						

* Arugula, Cilantro, Corn Salad, Cress, Mesclun
** Malabar, New Zealand

████████ sow seeds directly in garden
▒▒▒▒▒▒▒▒ sow seeds or plant transplants directly in garden
||||||||||||| plant transplants directly in garden

Chart provided courtesy of Sarah Strombeck-Charlesworth in conjunction with the Brooklyn Botanic Garden.

Once you find your region's chart, identify which foods you actually eat. Don't grow stuff you don't know what to do with or you'll be faced with two learning curves at once, one in the garden and a second in the kitchen. Go easy on yourself, and don't bite off more than you can chew.

permaculture 101

Permaculture is a way of setting up your living and growing space so that it mimics natural systems. Don't worry, you needn't move into a yurt and bathe in the nearby stream; the key word is *mimics*. All this really means is, use common sense, utilize all the resources at hand (wind, gravity, light, old yogurt containers, whatever), and strive for efficiency (i.e., minimize how much you're going to have to work or pay).

As with all the ideas in this chapter, permaculture is an entire movement and has an oeuvre to match. Looking up Bill Mollison and David Holmgren is a good way to start delving into the principles in more depth.

You might have heard about permaculture's bedfellow, biodynamic farming, which focuses on no-waste, efficient farming by utilizing animals and techniques like pasture rotation so natural processes do most of the work. This is Joel Salatin's farm model, described in Michael Pollan's *The Omnivore's Dilemma* (required reading).

When it comes to urban permaculture, scale is everything. You probably aren't working with an orchard in your apartment scenario; don't worry, smaller is way better. Start by figuring out what you have.

homework: lie around

I learned in my permaculture design studies that the best way to become acquainted with your surroundings is to lie around (hammock preferred) and observe them as the day progresses. See how the sun angles and ambles its way across the sky; see where you have direct sunlight.

Notice the slope of the ground. Are there any agents at work in your ecosystem—birds, bugs, bees? Do you have access to water? How far away is the compost pile? If you're planning a raised garden bed, will it be a pain in the ass to unload soil into your plot?

Black thumbs of the world, don't worry. By setting yourself up using nature as your guide (instead of viewing it as the thing to overcome), you're making failure nearly impossible.

toxic or uninspired soil

Testing your soil is a good idea, especially in urban areas with old buildings (or in new construction areas, since you might not know what was there before you and your house). Lead and mercury are common heavy metals found in urban soil, and petroleum leaches into and lingers in soils. Call your local university extension office (where you might get a heavy metal test kit for free) or visit your local nursery or hardware store for a soil test kit.

word to the wise

Buy plant starts for plants that are not direct-seeded (i.e., planted directly in the ground or an outside container) if you live in a cave-like dwelling or you'll become a slave to grow-light-innovation-on-the-fly and seedling-salvaging efforts.

Yes, it's more expensive (since a seed packet is about $2.50 and a single plant start is anywhere between $3-6), but urban, small-plot gardeners will rarely use all the seeds in a packet, and you run the risk of not storing them properly for future years' use. If you're growing in containers, you probably don't have enough room for more than three tomato plants, anyway.

93

Even if your garden soil isn't toxic, it may be too acidic or alkaline, excessively packed, or too sandy or clayey, or maybe it's just incapable of hosting plant life. You have two choices (neither of which is scrapping the idea of planting a garden):

- Amend it with organic fertilizer and compost (and patience). Certain plants also take up toxins from soils (but must be disposed of carefully).
- Build up right away and let a couple years of raised beds do the work of amending the soil for you.

raised garden beds

Raised beds are an ideal solution to imperfect, uninspired, or excessively compacted soil. By building up, you get to start growing things immediately, and after a few years of nurturing, the soil below will benefit from a trickle-down effect, thus making it a richer and deeper source of nutrients for your plants. You can plop the structure for a raised bed down wherever you please. The only drawback is that you'll need to get your hands on a bunch of good-quality garden soil to fill it. Ask a friend with a pickup truck to take you to the local plant nursery, and offer to feed him or her something homemade and yummy in return. (Sending your friend home with a loaf of homemade bread might boost your chances of having him or her answer the phone next time your number appears on your friend's caller ID.)

build your own raised bed

Gardens are great for building relationships between yourself and your surroundings (including neighbors). When I lived in

Austin, Texas, I built my 4-foot-by-4-foot raised bed atop a gangly patch of crabgrass that also happened to butt right up to my residential neighborhood curb. As I dug and pulled up as much of the crabgrass as I could (crabgrass is a real bitch), my garden project garnered a bunch of strange looks. The curbside location was not selected as a means of showing-off my vegetables; I hadn't enough sun anywhere else.

You'll need:

- Two 2-inch-by-8-inch-by 8-feet planks (have your hardware store saw them both in half, so you end up with four planks that are 4 feet long each). This is a great time to graduate from those punk rock cinder-block-and-board bookcases (noted in Chapter 2), since you can repurpose your planks as garden bed walls, like I did.
- Four (or eight, if you want to doubly reinforce) corner brackets, with screws
- Cardboard (to control grass or other invasive weeds below your plot)
- Half a cubic yard of soil (100 gallons) to fill the bed

Mel Bartholomew's *Square Foot Gardening* has an excellent photo tutorial on how to build a raised bed (and creative garden problem solving in general). I've never added the grid or bottom panel as he suggests, and I've still enjoyed full harvests.

battling the bugs

The kinds of bugs your plants attract is the best way to know what's going on. I went to my local nursery in my first year of garden tending with questions for a staff member about a mysterious spinach invader. She told me that the bugs in my case meant the plant was in distress, and with due cause; I was two months past the spinach growing season. I should've already pulled them up and composted. No wonder!

GOOD BUGS

- Ladybugs
- Roly poly bugs
- Spiders
- Earthworms
- Bees and wasps

BOTHERSOME BUGS

I won't get into the details of all the pesky little buggers you might encounter, but here's a list of common pests to prompt your Google Images search:

- Mealybugs
- Scales
- Aphids
- Spider mites
- White flies
- Caterpillars

After you identify your pest, treat the plant or soil accordingly. Home remedies are the best (and cheapest) way to solve your pest problems. I like the variety of recipes featured on Austin's own The Natural Gardener website, naturalgardeneraustin.com, which can be used for issues you'll encounter in any region, not just Central Texas.

compost: eew or ooh

So what is compost, anyway, and why shouldn't you be afraid to touch it? Let me start by saying that you touch germier things every single day, like subway rails, door handles, ATMs, the

ladybug

earthworm

phone receiver in your office, and elevator buttons. You're still alive, right?

When you turn to toxic chemicals, like commercial disinfectants or bleach, you kill everything involved, including the good bacteria and other microbes that assist our bodies. Read up on the "hygiene hypothesis" and maybe reconsider antibacterializing everything you encounter. Whether or not you accept this hypothesis—the idea that since our immune systems don't have much going on these days (that is, they aren't called upon to fight off common bacterial infections as often), our ultraclean environments are actually enhancing allergic reactions to common things like mold, animal dander, pollen, dust and dust mites, and certain foods—at least get the toxic stuff out of your home. Check in with Chapter 5 for homemade, nontoxic cleaning alternatives.

Okay, swinging back from my mini-rant/tangent: compost. Using your own food and yard waste is the very best you can do by your plants. Not only is it efficient, but it's also better than pitching food scraps and decomposing refrigerator matter into your indoor trash can, which makes it develop that hideous smell and also clutters up landfills unnecessarily.

The cool thing about nature's way of managing decomposition is that it involves a ton of bacteria, fungi, and insects doing the thing they do best: eat. The food chain that is decomposition (which in turn makes for fantastic soils) is a giant

quick fix

Make a simple soapy water mix by diluting a few drops of dish soap or Dr. Bronner's liquid soap (unscented is perfectly fine, but peppermint and lavender oils are known insect repellents) into a spray bottle filled with water and apply directly to foliage; this manages most of the pests listed here.

97

cleaning and balancing process. When your bugs and microbes have done their jobs, you scoop out a crumbly, earthy-smelling handful of stuff that you could actually eat (again). (I recommend feeding it to your plants, though.)

indoor/outdoor composting setups

Our countertop compost collector is a simple glass cookie jar stashed out of direct view in the corner near the sink. You can hide your compost jar under the kitchen sink or in an easily accessible cupboard if the jar creeps you out. When it gets full, we dump it into our 11-cubic-foot compost bin outside. The outdoor bin has a lid, air vents, and a handy bottom hatch for scooping out the best kind of black gold anyone can make.

Yeah, you can be crafty and make your own bin, but the $90–$120 investment in a backyard bin is well worth it. It's easy. You can't mess it up. It won't smell (if you add the right kinds and proportions of browns and greens). The animals that aren't supposed to be in there can't get in. And you don't *really* have to turn it. (Turning your compost pile every couple of weeks helps microbes and larger bugs thrive by incorporating the greens with the browns and distributing heat and moisture evenly.)

Do as you wish; there are a zillion ways to assemble a DIY compost pile setup, and plenty of books to help you identify solutions to your specific composting situations. Check out these books to answer all your compost questions:

- *Teaming with Microbes: The Organic Gardener's Guide to the Soil Food Web*
- *The Rodale Book of Composting: Easy Methods for Every Gardener*

THE HIP GIRL'S GUIDE TO HOMEMAKING

greens versus browns

There are two basic kinds of materials you want to populate your compost pile: "greens" for nitrogen and "browns" for carbon.

Greens should constitute 40 percent of your pile:

- Kitchen scraps (no oils, meat, or bones because they're harder for the microbes to break down and they'll attract pests)
- Cottonseed meal
- Garden wastes
- Pet (or human) hair
- Fresh grass clippings (pick up a neighbor's yard bag before the city does)

Browns make up the other 60 percent of your healthy compost pile:

- Coffee grounds
- Eggshells
- Stale flours, spices, and dry beans
- Shredded paper (not colored or shiny)
- Sawdust (also helps control smell and lower the temperature in a pile that's gotten too hot)
- Dry leaves, brown grass clippings
- Alfalfa hay or wheat straw

composting indoors

You still have compost options in your tiny, yardless apartment. Most farmers' markets and community gardens have a food scraps drop-off area, although there is a degree of

99

three tips for successful composting

1. Your compost pile actually needs some sunlight to thrive. Sunlight heats things up in there and activates decomposition.

2. Give the microbes a hand by keeping kitchen scraps smaller (and thus making them more easily digested). Crumble eggshells and dice tough fruit rinds or large vegetable scraps to keep your pile decomposing at a steady and even pace.

3. Place your compost bin where you can access it easily. The farthest corner of the yard is not automatically the best location for it, especially if you have a big yard.

impracticality involved: if you cook a lot, like we do, you're going to have way too many food scraps to conveniently carry on public transit (or your bike), and you'll need to do it at least once a week. (We empty our small countertop container two to three times a week.) Another issue I've run across is that in winter months, you might need to haul your scraps farther away, to some central location operated by either the city or an organic gardening association, since community gardens and markets aren't usually operating then.

Maybe you have a chest freezer? By all means, keep your scraps in there until you haul them off to the compost drop-off. Public compost pickup is becoming available in many cities, which is heartening because it cuts down on the bulk in already crowded landfills. If you don't live in Seattle, San Francisco, or Ann Arbor, where the city picks up your food scraps, then send a message to city council members and tell them you're interested in adding a public composting initiative. Two small towns in Massachusetts just introduced public compost pickup to the East Coast.

Your best bet for ridding your house of food wastes in small spaces is to investigate vermicomposting—composting with worms. This may be a little out there for you, but think about the benefits:

100

- It's a year-round solution.
- There's no smell.
- You can be flexible with temperatures, though room temp is best.
- Castings (aka worm poop) are jackpot assets in the garden.
- It requires only a utility closet or a small bin under your sink (which will fit nicely because you're going to get rid of all the chemical cleaning supplies after you read the next chapter.
- There's not a lot of work involved (on your part, at least).
- You can trade some of your compost "harvest" for friends' home-grown foods. I just swapped some of my watermelon rind pickles for a three-pound bag of worm castings.

Grab a copy of *Worms Eat My Garbage: How to Set Up and Maintain a Worm Composting System* or *The Urban Homestead* for DIY worm bin setups plus troubleshooting scenarios. Before you rush out for worms, go visit a friend who has a setup like this and see if it's going to work for you (i.e., to see if you get too grossed out).

five fun things to do with homegrown foods

1. Mojitos with your stoop-grown mint. Mint is the easiest thing to grow. Watch out, though; it has a mind of its own and spreads like crazy. Don't keep it near other plant pots or it'll invade.
2. Pesto with your window basil.

3. Super-small batches of preserves with strawberries or raspberries you grew on your fire escape.
4. Salads all summer long with your own lettuce mix.
5. Trading some of your produce for things you didn't grow but another friend did.

resources

Remember that your best resource is your local organic plant nursery. Your regional university extension office and local botanic garden are also great places to start for local planting guides, suggestions about plant varieties, and tips.

books

Great sources for information about methods:

- *Taylor's Guide to Houseplants* by Gordon P. Dewolf.
  An excellent primer on house and container plants.
- *Square Foot Gardening* by Mel Bartholomew.
  Creative use of minimal space, plus great photo tutorials for building your own raised beds.
- *The Urban Homestead* by Kelly Coyne and Erik Knutzen.
  Detailed how-tos on DIY projects.
- *Kitchen Harvest: A Cook's Guide to Growing Organic Fruit, Vegetables and Herbs in Containers* by Susan Berry.
  A not-too-involved primer focusing on edibles in containers, helpful for those of us who are spatially challenged.
- *You Grow Girl* by Gayla Trail.
  Great pictures of tricky things and an all-around, nonstressful guide to all things garden.

If you need inspiration:

- ⇢ *Animal, Vegetable, Miracle: A Year of Food Life* by Barbara Kingsolver (and family).
- ⇢ *The Omnivore's Dilemma* by Michael Pollan.

web

On the Web, try the following sites to build community and ask questions:

- ⇢ veggieharvest.com
- ⇢ hyperlocavore.ning.com
- ⇢ forums.gardenweb.com
- ⇢ naturalgardeneraustin.com
  Home remedies for pest control.
- ⇢ seedsavers.org
  Get heirloom seeds in the mail.

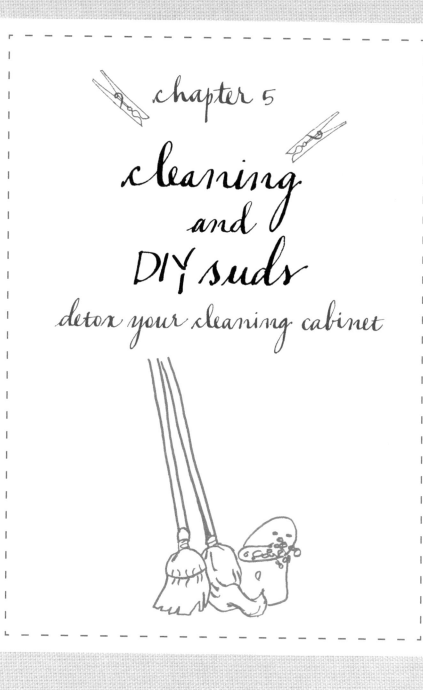

chapter 5

cleaning
and
DIY suds
detox your cleaning cabinet

I'm usually at odds with my house when it comes to cleaning. We have high-yield hair- and dust-producing pets. My house isn't dirty, it's just well lived in.

Cleaning is the vehicle to maintaining a space you enjoy that doesn't stress you out or make you sick. Most cleaning advisors swear by regular weekly cleaning schedules. We do our best around here, but it certainly isn't weekly or regular. The only routine cleaning I (barely) manage is doing the dishes (as you read in Chapter 1), cleaning the countertops and place mats after meals, and sweeping the floor when stuff sticks to my bare feet. I am not one to judge people based on their housekeeping.

For well-rounded advice, I phoned my friend Cassie to get input on some of the things I'm not interested in, like vacuuming. When I gasped at her admission that she vacuums every day and mops every three days or so, she aptly pointed out that everyone's situation is different and you should really do as little as you can get away with. She happens to have two small children, a firefighter husband (who always comes home covered in debris), and a constant stream of dirt from outdoor living, including a backyard chicken coop, a rope swing, and a kick-ass garden. Her cleaning schedule is based on necessity, not religion. Me, I don't have small children crawling around ingesting floor nasties left and right. I clean when my house grosses me out or when we're expecting guests. Hopefully you live with someone with a balanced notion of cleanliness to either trigger you into action more often or counteract your impulse to sterilize the house.

Cleaning is a momentum kind of thing for me. I'll get the urge to pull out the broom, and by the time I have dustpan in hand, I've coaxed myself into filling the sink with hot water and a few glugs of vinegar and grabbing the mop. (The sweeping-up part is usually the most time-consuming aspect anyway.) Tricking myself into productivity with treat incentives is particularly helpful in the housecleaning realm. For such toils I might earn an evening on the couch sipping a basil julep and watching *Mad Men* via Netflix.

This chapter covers some basics in the potentially perplexing realm of household toxins, with reference to cleaning supplies and why you don't really need to buy them at all. Commonsense cleaners like vinegar and baking soda might just show you once and for all that spending a bunch of money on cleaning supplies is throwing money down the toilet.

I'm not lying to you when I say that most homemade (or eco-friendly commercial products) cleaners work as effectively, if not better in some cases, than heavy-hitting chemicals, not to mention sparing you and your house from dangerous fumes.

mom knows best, or does she?

When it comes to what cleaning products to use, whom should you believe?

What your mom does/did is probably what you do. My mom has always cleaned with vinegar, luckily for me. She also taught me how to clean thoroughly and well—not just spreading dust and debris around, lifting things up, not cutting corners that will still need to be cleaned sometime.

Though I may not practice this skill set as often as I should, cleaning basics are one of the best things to impart to young people. Cleaning house with kid assistants is fun, though sometimes not the most efficient way, and you can conduct little lessons in chemistry (watch your drain fizz and react after you pour vinegar over baking soda) or morals (someone always has to clean up messes).

If you weren't as lucky as me, not to worry; I think old dogs can learn new tricks, especially if those tricks end up saving you a bunch of money.

toxic soup under your kitchen sink

I'm not trying to be all doom and gloom on your ass, but hear me out. First is the case for you, and second is the case for everyone else (aka the planet).

Making the case for you: The EPA has shown that indoor air is on average two to five times more polluted than air outside, even in urban areas. Cleaning supplies and air fresheners release the not-so-good kind of organic compounds while you are using them and, to some extent, when they are stored under sinks and in garages. Elevated concentrations of volatile organic compounds (VOCs, which you may remember from the section on bathroom paint jobs in Chapter 3) can persist in the home long after chemicals are sprayed or cleaning activities conclude.

Making the case for the planet: When you use products with harsh chemicals, we run into trouble as these things shoot down the drain and out into the water that we eventually drink, that we use to water our food crops, and that cycles into the atmosphere. The U.S. Geological Survey con-

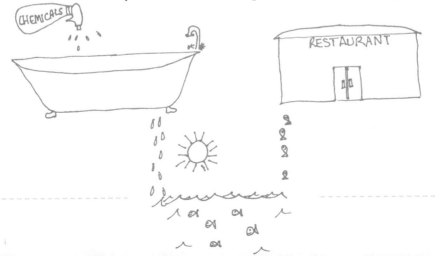

ducted a study in 2002, testing 139 streams across thirty states. They found that half of the streams contained seven or more chemicals in the following categories: steroids, insect repellants, caffeine, triclosan, detergent metabolites, and plasticizers like phthalates. Things you might

Word to the Wise

Beware of greenwashing! "Green" cleaners are not always green. As you've probably noticed, marketers are cunning, and certain products' labeling requirements are lax.

Check out my favorite truly ecofriendly brands in the "Resources" section at the end of this chapter for help deciphering the cleaning supply aisle.

not think twice about squirting onto your dishes or into the toilet bowl actually have the potential to affect fish reproduction or produce prolonged impacts on algae and bacterial life (which is, coincidentally, the basis for all other forms of life).

the secret life of chemicals

The guys who wrote the book *Slow Death by Rubber Duck: The Secret Danger of Everyday Things,* Rick Smith and Bruce Lourie, informed me that there are 82,000 chemicals in use in the United States, with 700 new ones added each year. Of these 82,000, only 650 are monitored through the EPA's Toxic Release Inventory and only 200 have ever been tested for toxicity.

Jaw drop is the obvious response. Those numbers alone should shock you into reading a few labels and understanding that the chemical industry is using us all as guinea pigs for new and exciting chemical cocktails.

Personally, I find the following aspects of suspected chemical pollutants rather sinister:

- No one knows for sure the long-term effects of chemicals that have marginal (or no) scientifically proven safety assessments. By subjecting ourselves to things that haven't been proven safe in long-term studies, we're increasing risk factors for developing cancer, autism, asthma, infertility, miscarriages, behavioral disorders, and even obesity.

- Toxic crap down the drain or in the landfill doesn't disappear, and most often it spreads out (via the food chain, affecting high-level predators, like ourselves, the most) or morphs into compounds that are even more dangerous or difficult for our bodies and planet to get rid of. Our bodies' fat cells and brain receptors make for nice storage units for toxins—gross! This pervasiveness affects not only ourselves but also future generations; not exactly the thing you were hoping to pass along to your kids.

- Using most commercial cleaning products increases your risk of accidentally encountering toxic combos. Mixing anything that contains chlorine bleach with something that includes ammonia or even vinegar has highly toxic consequences.

- Product manufacturers are not required to list all ingredients if they're part of a proprietary formula. Who knows what you're actually spraying all over your furniture and countertops?

- Commercial cleaning products (which, as you'll see you later in the chapter, you don't even need) are expensive. Who has extra money to dish out on biohazards?

label savvy

GOOD:

- ▸▸ Acetic acid is vinegar.
- ▸▸ Carbonic acid is in club soda.
- ▸▸ Citric acid is found in lemon juice.
- ▸▸ Sodium bicarbonate is baking soda.
- ▸▸ Sodium borate is borax.
- ▸▸ Sodium chloride is salt.

BAD:

- ▸▸ Sodium hydroxide is lye; it's highly corrosive and prevalent in drain and oven cleaners.
- ▸▸ Sodium hypochlorite is chlorine bleach.
- ▸▸ Ammonia is the active ingredient in most all-purpose cleaners and window/glass cleaners like Windex.

OKAY:

- ▸▸ Sodium carbonate is washing soda, which is one of the active ingredients in most laundry products; it's one of the most alkaline products you could use (by itself, it peels wax off flooring).
- ▸▸ Sodium perborate is sodium salt or perboric acid, an oxidizing agent commonly found in cleaning supplies.

There's actually good news on the takeaway, though. You're not going to go broke buying a

avoiding the three biggest household cleaning and maintenance toxins

1. Don't use synthetic air fresheners, sprays, plug-ins, etc. Pick up an essential oil diffuser if you can't go without.

2. Never buy liquid drain cleaners; instead, snake clogs loose. Drain cleaners are not effective in handling tough clogs, and they eat away at your pipes and muck up the watershed.

3. Forget oven cleaners. Use a baking soda paste for oven cleaning and skip your evening trip to the gym.

111

bunch of fancy eco-brand cleaning products; you're going to make your own. Discover a bunch of low-cost, effective cleaning solutions in the second half of the chapter.

germageddon:
hygiene hype or hypothesis?

You're either in one camp or the other on this one, exceedingly hygienic or a proponent of the ten-second rule as a way of building up immunity to the sixty thousand different types of germs you are likely to encounter on a daily basis. I started out in the latter group, migrated to the former, and then found my way back to my original camp. Now I'm somewhere in the middle. There is a lot of terrifying literature out there about germs, and it's hard to understand; it's also tough to make the necessary connections between cleaning supply industry giants and the scientists they are funding within academic institutions.

Eight simple things to help you make sense of cleaning product rhetoric, scientific studies, and basic chemistry:

1. Anything labeled "disinfectant" is a pesticide (and kills 99.9 percent of microorganisms, as required by the EPA to be so labeled).
2. A full 10 percent of your dry body weight is bacteria, some of which you couldn't live without.
3. Exposure to germs (both good and bad) does not automatically make you sick.
4. Your immune system is a powerful line of defense, so in most cases it's better to focus on keeping yourself healthy (and supporting your immune system) than to go on haphazard killing sprees around the house.

5. Applying science to the realities of the home is really just risk assessment and risk management—a fancy way of saying that you weigh the pros and cons and decide what's best for you under the circumstances.

6. Unless you're conducting surgeries or having people in your house with severely compromised immune systems (some elderly populations or those who are very ill), you're sterilizing to your own (and the planet's) detriment.

7. Sterility is impossible—germs travel in the air, and your house does not exist in a vacuum. (Many bacteria do their best work in a vacuum, by the way.)

8. You might lose sight of or interest in important things (like gardening, cooking, sex, or leaving the house) if you become too microbe-centric.

Read on to understand how to protect yourself from germs while coexisting with our microbial friends.

myth of sterilization

Not only is a sterile, germ-free house an unattainable venture, but attempting this doesn't do your house many favors in the long run. As I read *Good Germs, Bad Germs: Health and Survival in a Bacterial*

look for statements like these on the cleaning products you buy

- Plant-based
- Petroleum-free
- Nontoxic
- Biodegradable
- Non-bioaccumulative
- Cruelty-free
- No phosphates
- Fragrance-free or free of synthetic fragrances

113

word to the wise

Using chlorine bleach around your house creates a slew of particularly dangerous compounds called organochlorines, which are generally toxic, plus they cause cancer in animals and likely in humans. Thanks, but no thanks.

When you do need to disinfect, use a botanical disinfectant like Benefect or Seventh Generation's disinfecting products, which utilize an extract of thyme leaves to achieve the same EPA-certified kill rate as chlorine bleach.

World by Jessica Snyder Sachs, an apt statement struck me from her interviews with microbiologist David Thaler: "Whenever you make a sterile surface, you become a victim of whatever falls on it. It's like plowing a field and not planting anything but instead trying to live on whatever weeds happen to pop up."

The Washington Toxics Coalition provides a number of free fact sheets advising how good cleaning is much more important than disinfecting. Studies show that it's best to wash your hands frequently, especially before eating and after using the bathroom, and use proper kitchen and food safety practices to prevent disease.

When it comes to cleaning house, your best bet is to clean frequently handled objects periodically with soap and water or vinegar. Though vinegar isn't an EPA-registered disinfectant, my self-bestowed chemistry/microbiology degrees taught me that the acidity of vinegar does render inert (if not kill outright) most pathogens found in the home.

antibacterials, busted

Many of the antibacterial products in heavy circulation on our countertops and in our under-sink cupboards don't protect us from viruses or aren't used in the right capacity or concentration for the chemicals to be effective.

114

Stop spending money on antimicrobial-infused products like:

- Hand soaps
- Liquid dish soaps
- Aerosols (you can't disinfect the air, sorry)
- Toothpastes
- Clothing

Before buying any disinfecting or sanitizing products for your house, you should ask yourself if eliminating microbes is absolutely critical. Targeted disinfection is optimal for cases where food is involved or when there is someone with a delicate immune system; otherwise, clean regularly and stick with household cleaners like the homemade examples provided in the latter half of the chapter.

out with the old

Getting rid of the toxic cleaning cabinet mélange can be tricky. Type this into Google with your city or state name before it: "household hazardous waste disposal." Towns and local businesses often sponsor drop-offs for specific household hazardous items, like compact fluorescent bulbs, batteries, and old paint. You can also consult earth911 .com, using the term "HHW" where it asks "find recycling centers for" and your zip code, to find your nearest one.

Hip Trick

Keep your sponge, ditch the germs: boil your sponge for at least three minutes (and follow by microwaving it for two minutes if you want). *Cook's Illustrated* magazine (January-February 2003) found this method reduced the bacteria count most and was twice as effective as soaking the sponge in a bleach solution.

Depending on your municipality's waste plan, you might be faced with tough decisions for ridding toxins from your house. Appallingly enough, I discovered that there are no HHW disposal sites that take toxic household cleaning supplies in my county. Giving away unused portions of products or carefully wrapping them before placing them in the regular trash is usually the best choice if HHW disposal isn't accessible to you.

in with the new

Once you get the bad stuff out (and deal with the potentially nightmarish method for doing so), make sure you don't need to deal with that experience again. Populating your under-sink area with the following cleaning ingredients will keep you and your home safe and healthy.

The awesome threesome:

- **Vinegar** is a low-cost, effective resource for killing most mold, bacteria, and germs due to its acidity level. I use it to clean just about everything in my house: wood floors, kitchen floor, countertops after food prep, even mirrors and windows. The Food and Drug Administration (FDA) specifically mentions its effectiveness in reducing populations of household bacteria and germs. Distilled white vinegar is what you want; save your cider and other vinegars for eating and pickling.
- **Baking soda** is your go-to for stuck-on stuff, be it food crusted stubbornly into

116

a pot, soap scum on your tub, or old cooking experiments gone wrong in your oven. Baking soda also doubles as a deodorizer, which you probably already know since you likely have an open box in your fridge right now.

❧ **Dish soap** cleans everything else.

Yes, you read that right. The stuff that's sitting on the side of your sink right now can pick up the slack where vinegar and baking soda didn't work. Wash your car, your stained concrete floors, and your granite countertops with a squirt of dish soap in a bucket or sink filled with water.

what the heck is distilled white vinegar anyway?

The fermentation process (which is really just the controlled use of microorganisms, in this case yeast) breaks corn down into ethanol (alcohol), water, and carbon dioxide. The liquids are then distilled to separate the ethanol from the water. The alcohol is then aerated so that *Acetobacter* bacteria will consume the alcohol and convert it to acetic acid, which is vinegar.

If you have the option next time you're at the store, grab white vinegar that touts its non-GMO (not genetically modified) status. The others are made with corn from farms all across America, which happens to be 60 percent GMO, according to the USDA. It'll be a little more expensive, but not as expensive as the chemical cleaners a few aisles over.

other good ingredients to have on hand

- **Simple suds** like castile soap (which is not a detergent like dish soap) is useful for cleaning bodies and hands, pretreating laundry stains, and pest control in the garden. We buy the gallon jug of Dr. Bronner's and refill our hand soap pumps and shower bottle as needed.

- **Salt** can be used as an abrasive in boosting baking soda's might in cleaning tough-to-remove food from counters, sinks, and pans or as a drain deodorizer.

- **Lemon juice** is one of the strongest food acids, effective against most household bacteria, and a sweet-smelling bleach alternative in laundry you plan to hang dry in the sun. I like to do periodic lemon juice and salt scrubs (followed by a suntanning session) for our cutting board.

- **Hydrogen peroxide** is a safer sanitizing and oxidizing agent than chlorine bleach and can be used for whitening everything from your teeth to the toilet bowl.

- **Borax** is where to turn when you need more alkaline oomph than baking soda, like in the case of overgrown mold and mildew. It's super potent stuff (though not harmful for the environment or you when used properly), so you'll want to wear gloves if you're scrubbing with it.

- **Essential oils** are a dee-luxe ingredient that can be added to any of your homemade recipes to make you feel like you're cleaning with fancy products. I love adding lavender, bergamot, or orange oil to vinegar or baking soda solutions. Pure essential oils (not blends) are great ways to infuse your cleaning supplies with in-scent-ives for getting the job done.

- **Citrus solvent** products like Citra Solv base their cleaning muscle on a citrus oil extract called d-limonene, which should only be used on the toughest of jobs. We use Citra Solv to degrease and degunk our stovetop burners during our seasonal deep clean.

tools on deck

Don't go buy a bunch of crap. You don't need most of it.

Essentials:

- Broom
- Dustpan and dust brush duo
- Sponges with scrubber sides (old kitchen sponges are perfect because they won't scratch surfaces)
- Kitchen sink drain plug or bucket
- Two decent spray bottles (reused eco-product bottles are fine; I advise not reusing any bottle that contained bleach- or ammonia-laced products since they create potent reactions with other ingredients)
- Rags

inspiring cleaning ideas from hip girl's blog readers

- Catch up on podcasts or favorite radio shows while you clean.
- Blast the radio or your stereo and rock out.
- Put on your cleaning shoes; some readers mentioned wearing special sneakers to get in the mood.
- Polish the floor in a pair of old, thick socks and get a twofer: an excuse to dance around plus a shiny floor! (Just watch your toes around the bed frame!)
- Scrubbing builds arm muscles and increases strength over time. The more you clean, the more toned you'll be!

119

Don't buy cleaning rags. Your house produces plenty of rag-worthy stuff. Downcycle those bathroom linens that have seen better days. Promote lone-ranger socks, the ones whose mates have long since left them, to a cleaning post by cutting them open to make a flat rag. Tear up old T-shirts for excellent cleaning/dusting/buffing cloths. If you insist on buying a matching stack, grab a bundle of 100 percent cotton towels at a kitchen supply store.

vacuum power

I don't own a vacuum because I don't have carpet.

My best friend, Cassie, doesn't have carpet, yet she owns a vacuum. She has a high-action household (as mentioned in the introduction to this chapter) and vacuums every day to make sure she's on the winning side of the dust and debris battle. Plus she likes knowing that what's entering her children's mouths is mostly from the kitchen table.

As it should be with anything you touch every day, you know Cassie loves the hell out of her vacuum. Her mother bestowed upon her a Miele vacuum as a birthday gift, and life as she knew it changed drastically. A fancy sweeper machine, like a turbo-powered stand mixer, is something you might have to reserve for parental gifts, wedding (or milestone birthday) registries, or winning the lottery.

If Miele is not in your forecast anytime soon, look for any HEPA-filtered vacuum. Most non-HEPA vacuums spray dust particles around the house and cause allergen levels to rise because the filter bags are inefficient.

housecleaning without a calculator

Dilution could very well be the trickiest part of DIY cleaning supplies. The good news is that (unlike with chemical cleaning dilutions) you really can't mess up with DIY dilutions. You may end up using more of something than you actually need, but nothing in your nontoxic cleaning cabinet will burn holes through anything if used at a stronger dilution than necessary.

Should you find yourself interested in precision, then figure out the volume of whatever you usually use to clean: your kitchen sink, your handy bucket, your spray bottle. Nail the volume breakdown of a gallon to your forehead: 1 gallon = 4 quarts = 8 pints = 16 cups =128 fluid ounces.

When reading dilution instructions, you'll often see ratios like 1:4, which means 1 part product to 4 parts water. For 1 gallon of concentrate, this means 128 fl oz divided by 4, which yields 32 fl oz. So 1 quart (32 fl oz) of product was added to 4 quarts (128 fl oz) of water.

making the switch

I don't spend a lot of time making cleaning supplies. I rarely take the time to put together the cleaning product recipes in the two fantastic books I own (though putting a few drops of essential oil in a box of baking soda or a spray bottle filled with half water and half vinegar is technically following a recipe).

The first time you clean with something as basic as vinegar, you might feel like you're not really cleaning. Now that you're hip to how all these things work, you can let go of the need for suds-

Hip Trick

Tear a cotton ball in half, dot it with real vanilla extract (not the faux stuff), and suck it up like regular debris the next time you use your vacuum. You'll infuse the house with a sweet smell while you clean!

ing bubbles, which you'll see in Chapter 6 are just for show. Bidding bubbles and bleach good-bye can be tough, so if one clean sweep feels intimidating, start by phasing out certain kinds of cleaners. Try implementing a few of the following suggestions until you realize you'd rather buy more fruit at the farmers' market than a bunch of expensive cleaners on a regular basis.

clean your whole house for 60¢

Get up right now. Grab your new spray bottle, fill it halfway with vinegar, and fill it the rest of the way with water. Add 5–10 drops of your favorite essential oil if the smell of vinegar is too much for you. This is pretty much the only thing you need to clean your whole house, bathroom to countertops.

Label the bottle if you want, but in our house we only have one unmarked spray bottle—this one—so we know what's in it.

drain duty

- Give your drains a regular monthly cleaning (or whenever you think of it) by pouring ½ cup baking soda down the drain and letting it sit for five minutes. Follow this with ½ cup vinegar down the drain. Cover the drain tightly for a few minutes while the fizz cleans your drains and pipes. Flush with cold water.
- Catch clogs early on by looking for slow drainage. Most clogs can be handled with a trusty plunger. If that doesn't do the job, it means

Hip Trick
Fill the rinse aid compartment of your dishwasher with plain white vinegar to keep spots from forming on dishes as they dry.

you have a deep clog and you'll need to snake it. In either case, toxic drain cleaners won't solve the problem; you'll just pollute the watershed.

stovetop scenarios

- Regularly wipe down the stove. If it's easy enough, lift up your burners and clean up after rice boils over or oil splatters while frying. Adding additional layers of grime with tomorrow's pancakes won't make stains any easier to remove.
- Seasonally soak your burners overnight in a citrus solvent to remove persistent sludge. This is especially necessary if you've been infected with the canning and preserving bug. Wear gloves and use a scrubby sponge in the morning to clean off all the sludge.
- Slosh around a splash of white vinegar in a stainless steel pot or pan suffering from the cloudy mineral deposits that appear after long-cooking projects, like rice.
- Use a clean rag or paper towel (this is the only thing we use paper towels for in our house) to clean your cast iron skillet after mild use. Grease and oil residue are the best way to season your skillet. This will also prevent food from sticking in the future.

  For really gunky clean-ups, either use kosher salt and a clean sponge or go ahead and use soap to cut some of the grease. Rinse the skillet well and place it on the burner over low heat to make sure no water remains or you'll find rust in the morning. Drop in and spread around about a teaspoon of any kind of oil

123

after it's dry. An aluminum pie tin makes a perfect lid for our 8-inch cast iron skillet, which we keep on the stovetop to accommodate daily use.

oven mishaps

➻ Make a baking soda paste by adding water until the baking soda is spreadable.

Spread the paste on oven surfaces. Let it sit overnight if it's really gross in there. Rub crusties off with a scrubby sponge, fine steel wool, and maybe a putty knife. Add salt to your sponge for extra scrubbing oomph. After scrubbing, spritz with your vinegar/ water spray bottle and wipe to remove any baking soda residue.

odors

➻ Spritz with your vinegar/water spray bottle.
➻ Use baking soda, dry or in a paste.
➻ Place a cotton ball soaked in vanilla extract or dotted with your fave essential oil in the problem area.
➻ Put a plate or saucer of fresh ground coffee in the smelly spot.

tub and shower tiles

➻ Spraying regularly with vinegar and water will inhibit mold and mildew.

- Use baking soda or borax pastes to scrub off established mold and mildew. Leave the paste on overnight if it's really bad.
- Spray persistent mildew with hydrogen peroxide and let it air dry. Peroxide is a natural disinfectant that will stop the spread of mildew, which will otherwise multiply profusely and take over your cave-like bathroom. Disinfecting in this case is necessary, so just be sure to use a product that's not going to leave lingering chemicals in your shower for you to inhale every time you're in there. Revisit Chapter 3 for tips on staying calm if you have a mildew situation.

mirrors, sinks, and windows

- Use your vinegar/water spray bottle to spray surfaces. For streak-free windows, wipe clean with a couple of sheets of scrunched up newspaper. Use one that's printed using soy-based ink so you don't release the nasty chemicals in synthetic inks.
- Use a clean coffee filter in place of newspaper if you're not sure about the ink.

toilet

- Flush your toilet and turn off the water (with the valve behind the toilet) before it has a chance to refill the bowl. Pour in a few glugs of vinegar and let it sit for a few minutes while you clean the rim, seat, and lid with your vinegar/water spray bottle. Pour in some baking

125

soda for extra scrubbing action and use your toilet brush as usual. Turn water back on and rinse off the brush as the toilet fills.

One of the microbiologists I interviewed said that thinking your toilet will ever be sterile is just silly; clean it regularly and you'll be fine. (I venture to extend that thinking to the rest of the house.)

floors:
wood, linoleum, tile

- Fill a bucket and add 1 cup vinegar for every gallon of water
- Baking soda paste handles scuffs.
- A squirt of dish soap in your bucket or sink filled with water can be used for things you don't want to subject to the acidity of vinegar (concrete, granite or marble, newly finished wood flooring).

resources

safe cleaning product brands

- Biokleen
- Citra Solv
- Dr. Bronner's
- Earth Friendly Products (Dishmate line)
- Ecover
- Seventh Generation

books

- *Better Basics for the Home: Simple Solutions for Less Toxic Living* by Annie Berthold-Bond.
  A comprehensive guide to home cleaning with nontoxic ingredients, plus great info on how to make your own personal care products using only a handful of ingredients.
- *Clean House, Clean Planet* by Karen Logan.
  Great source for tons of house cleaning recipes to try in different scenarios.
- *Good Germs, Bad Germs* by Jessica Snyder Sachs.
  Geek out over microbes and understand how our bodies thrive with microbial assistance. This might make you reconsider (or at least delay) Germageddon and possibly run to the store for probiotics.
- *Slow Death by Rubber Duck* by Rick Smith and Bruce Lourie.
  Smart and interesting read on how to make sense of a confusing world of products and potential (and proven) health hazards.

web

- Find your nearest household hazardous waste disposal by zip code: earth911.com.
- Search the EPA's chemical database to understand what's in your cleaning products: epa.gov.
- Ask Science Man any questions you have about cleaning with nontoxic ingredients or products: seventh generation.com/learn/ask-science-man.

127

- Read excellent, free publications on sustainability from the Washington Toxics Coalition: watoxics.org /publications.
- Look for products that hold up to true ecofriendly standards: greenseal.org.

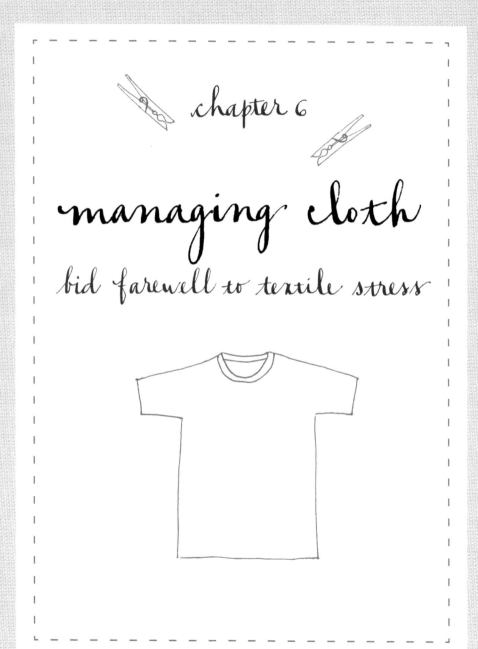

chapter 6

managing cloth

bid farewell to textile stress

Cloth gets its own chapter because it's a beastly chore. There's no avoiding it for too long. You have to wear clothes. You have to dry your hands. You have to sleep on sheets.

I'm clumsy, and I've come to terms with the fact that I'll be wearing some remnant of whatever I'm eating or drinking. Plus the bane of my existence is the stacks of cloth lying around: the mending pile and the hand-wash-only stack. There's no convenient place for them, and as the piles get bigger, my stress level increases.

In this chapter I've experimented with nontoxic stain treatment and laundering. Admittedly, I care about the watershed and whether future generations will have enough to drink and use, but really, all these "specially formulated" laundering supplies are pretty expensive and we're on a strict budget. So allow me to offer some better suggestions.

Through my many washing experiments, I found that a squirt of dish soap or club soda usually handled stains best when they happened, and other home remedies handled the ones I didn't get to in time. Because I rely upon the launderette and a friend with a car to do laundry, I've got pretreating down. I do envy those just-throw-it-in-the-wash-right-away people, but sometimes weeks elapse between me and the borax-filled afternoon that is our little Brooklyn launderette.

As for mending, you could quite possibly know more about this task than I do, which will be a great opportunity for you to feel good about yourself. My mending motto is to just wing it. If you mess up, a few snips offer an instant undo. I don't love needle and thread, so I'm not going to force myself into excessive craftiness. I stick with basic hand sewing and manage just fine for my needs.

You'll also find a few simple cloth craft projects at the end of the chapter that even the most uncoordinated among us can manage.

making sense of scents

Later in this chapter you'll read about why you should be using detergents made with vegetable-derived surfactants, but let's start off with stinky stuff, which is a common lurker in laundry products.

My problem with most of the products out there, even some of the ecofriendly brands, is synthetic fragrance. Beyond the fact that aerosolized perfume particles can make their way into your lungs (gross), there's a fine balance between pleasantly infused and I-can't-get-far-enough-away-from-it. Most fragrances—if you're lucky enough to get an ingredient list—are synthetic (the ones listed as "fragrance" or "parfum") and derived from petrochemicals.

Phthalates, the petrochemicals commonly found in fragrance, are neurotoxic, which means they could interfere with brain function and change the way your receptors work over time. Not cool. (Like you needed another reason to be grossed out over your overly fragranced seatmate on the plane or bus, or that godawful plug-in scent diffuser at your aunt Judy's house.) Don't freak out, though—phthalate contaminants generally pass through your system within twelve hours. Give Aunt Judy an essential oil diffuser as an early birthday present and focus your energies on identifying and trying to reduce repeated exposures. Read more about how to give synthetic scents the boot in *Slow Death by Rubber Duck*.

In the meantime, don't worry: you aren't destined to a life devoid of scent. Revisit Chapter 5 for information on enjoying scented things based on pure essential oils, not synthetics.

131

the lowdown on laundry

Everyone's scenario is likely to be a little different. I met a bunch of people in college who hadn't the slightest idea what to do in the laundry room besides throw clothes in the hamper. I've been doing my own laundry since age twelve because I found it difficult to put away my clean, folded clothes after my mom took the time to wash them. When she discovered still folded, clean clothes at the bottom of my dirty clothes hamper, I got my first lesson on the throes of laundering.

A few reasons to consider doing your own laundry (as opposed to the drop-off service):

- Same deal as why you'd want to eat at home: you'll never find as high-quality components used by others as you can choose to use yourself. Laundries are businesses; they must keep costs low to make money. I can say with near certainty that they're not using Seventh Generation products, or if they are, you can bet you're ultimately paying double what you would for a bottle at the grocery store.
- Do you really want someone else folding your underwear?
- You made the stain, so presumably you know what to look for before it hits the dryer, which will set the stain.

friend dates

Ritualize and spice things up by doing laundry with a pal (for those of you non-in-house launderers). My friend and I frequent a launderette a couple of neighborhoods out of the way based entirely on the fact that this place is extra spacious, has a parking lot (a big deal in NYC), and sells both snacks and ice cream from vending machines.

We chat about work, dramas, cute clothes that emerge from each other's bags. We eat chips during the spin cycle and catch up on the many things that are going on in the context of our busy lives. All of these things are possible to conduct at any launderette.

the basics: laundry play-by-play

1. **Sort your clothes.** I always have enough dirty clothes to fill two or three separate loads. If you don't have that many, don't worry. You can wash most dark and light things together in cold water. The exception to this is known bleeders (like my kitchen rugs or magenta summer skirt). My standard loads are:

   - *Whites*
   - *Dark colors*
   - *What doesn't go in either of the above categories*

   This is also a good time to turn items right side out. A scrunched-up or balled-up sock won't get as clean as if it had all possible surface area exposed in the cycle.

2. **Choose your water temperature and load size.** Cold! Washing your clothes on the cold water setting not only saves you money on utility bills but keeps your clothes in good shape longer. Warm and hot water washes don't get your clothes any cleaner. Many

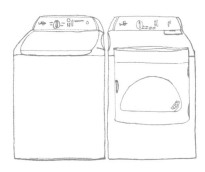

sources and studies show how hot water kills germs and dust mites, but your washing machine may not actually provide water hot enough to do the job. The same allergens and germs are more likely to die in the heated dryer or out on the line with a little help from UV rays.

Most detergents (both ecofriendly and regular commercial brands) are formulated now to work as well in cold water as in warm water, which formerly was the only way to make detergents work in hard water conditions. Plus colder wash temperatures are better for the planet, reducing carbon emissions by nearly a third for each load, and promoting the conservation of petroleum stocks.

3. **Choose your detergent.** First off, a liquid detergent will cut your carbon footprint in the laundry room by a third (because it takes more energy to make solid and powdered detergents). Look for concentrated detergents. Using less soap is better for your pocketbook and the planet.

Your laundry detergent's cleaning power is based on surfactants, and probably also includes enzymes and builders to help the surfactants work better. Most *surfactants* (both plant- and petroleum-derived) have the same basic structure: a hydrophobic (fat-loving) "tail" that binds to and mobilizes stain and soil particles, and a hydrophilic (water-loving) "head" that flushes the soil/surfactant duo out with the wastewater in the washing machine. (Just to be clear, a plant-derived surfactant detergent doesn't clean better or differently; I'd just rather use less petroleum in the process of washing my clothes.)

Enzymes are usually naturally occurring, but the

what's the difference between liquid soap, dish soap, and laundry detergent?

All three contain surfactants, or surface-active agents, which both attract dirt and repel it from fabric (or other surfaces in the case of dishes).

Liquid soaps are made from lye and a fat or oil; the former is very alkaline and the latter is very acidic, leaving soap with a slightly alkaline pH. Soaps base their cleaning power on glycerin, which helps oil mix with water. In pure castile soaps, like Dr. Bronner's, only vegetable oils (palm, coconut) were used to derive the glycerin.

Dish soap and laundry detergents have additional ingredients that boost their ability to dissolve oils (which surround stains) and let the surfactants do their job at shaking loose stains.

ones in your detergent are engineered via fermentation in laboratories to meet industrial demand levels. These biological helpers are just like the substances that break down food in your body. There are three main types of enzymes you'll find in laundry detergents:

- *Proteases help to break down proteins*
- *Lipases help to break down fat*
- *Amylases help to break down starches*

Builders serve in detergents to remove calcium and magnesium ions from wash water, helping the surfactant to

like you needed another reason not to use chlorine bleach . . .

Using bleach in your laundry load will kill the trusty enzymes in your detergent, which is more than you probably bargained for.

Word to the Wise

Steer clear of a combined color load with things you haven't ever washed since they might bleed. Test fabrics by getting a corner wet and squeezing it out; if color bleeds out into your sink, you should hand-wash.

do its job better. Additives, like borax and baking soda, work in a similar capacity by increasing alkalinity and thus the effectiveness of your detergent.

Choosing a larger load size than necessary for the amount of clothes you have will not improve the cleaning power of your wash. If you don't cram the clothes in too tightly, more clothes in the washer means better cleaning, because more friction is better than less. Towels are excellent at generating friction with their general heft.

4. **Add materials and pretend you're a mad scientist.** Since you probably just finished Chapter 5, you already have a keen sense of the magical properties of vinegar, baking soda, hydrogen peroxide, and borax. Those four wonder cleaners also help your laundry detergent perform better and eliminate the need for bad-for-you/bad-for-the-planet things like dryer sheets and chlorine bleach. In fact, our good friend borax is the star of the show in your laundry room.

Start with Seventh Generation laundry detergent, or another product with plant- (not petroleum-) derived surfactants, and experiment away. Here are my favorite laundry recipes:

Whites. For the brightest whites ever, add ½ cup borax to the wash cycle and then ¼ cup hydrogen peroxide to the rinse cycle (when you hear or see the water start going again after the wash cycle has finished). If you have the ability (i.e., your washer is in your home), once the tub is filled with rinse water stop the washer and let the clothes soak in the peroxide solution for a whitening boost.

Dark colors. Add ½ cup baking soda to the wash and the recommended amount of a color-safe, non-chlorine bleach like Seventh Generation's Free & Clear.

Other colors. Add ½ cup borax to the wash cycle and ¼–½ cup vinegar to the rinse cycle.

Don't worry, your clothes won't smell like any of the additives after the cycle is finished (even vinegar, I promise)!

static cling

I haven't used dryer sheets in two years, and nothing comes out static clingy.

Static cling happens in clothing when one surface is rubbed against another, causing a transfer of electrons; as a result, some clothes become positively charged and others become negatively charged. Synthetic fibers are especially prone to static cling because they don't absorb a lot of water (unlike wool or cotton), and humidity reduces the buildup of static electricity. Overdrying clothes in a tumble dryer will guarantee a shocking load of hot laundry.

Adding vinegar to the rinse cycle of your laundry is a great

word to the wise

Bubbles do not signal more intense cleaning; bubbles are really just for show.

Adding more detergent than you need (especially with highly concentrated detergents, which includes most brands on the market) will negatively impact cleaning and make your clothes look dingy, a result of excess detergent residue.

I cringe after seeing other machines at the launderette that are solid white with bubbles, so much so that you can't even see the clothes spinning around in there.

alternative to dryer sheets. If you enjoy the fresh scent provided by chemical-laden dryer sheets, drop a muslin teabag filled with dried lavender (packed full and tied tightly so no little flower buds escape) into the dryer with your wet clothes. You can use the same sachet for up to ten loads of drying.

stains

If you're enjoying your life, stains happen. You can either cover all surfaces in plastic (shudder) or enlighten yourself on pretreating so you can live like a normal person and remove the happy life stains when they inevitably happen.

Now that you've draped your table, towel racks, and maybe your kids and pets with the prettiest of pretties, here's what happens when life disrespects your decorating:

- It's wine night and you have intricate baby blue napkins.
- Your helpful friend cleaned up dog puke with your cute, gauzy towel (gee . . . thanks).
- Kids dropped the fruits of their labor on the kitchen table: potatoes (and worms) dug up from the garden.

Hip Trick
If you forgot about or didn't catch a stain early on, dampen the area with cold water and rub in a little squirt of dish soap to loosen the oils surrounding your stain before you wash it.

not all happy life stains are created equal

Nothing, to my knowledge (even the commercial, chemical stuff) is an all-purpose stain remover. Detergents try hard to be all-in-one stain busters, but you'll have to get to know your stain to understand what will be your best bet for removing it.

Here's a chart to help you get fresh with your stains:

TYPE OF STAIN	MY FAVORITE APPROACH	OTHER THINGS TO TRY
Oil, grease, lipstick	Dampen affected area and work in a dab of liquid soap (glycerin-based) in small circles. Add a sprinkle of baking powder to increase friction and loosen the stain. Rinse.	Sub a few drops of laundry detergent for the liquid soap in my favorite approach. For extra stain-busting power, soak in white vinegar or dab with concentrated Citra Solv.
Protein stains: blood, chocolate, coffee, mustard, mud, food, fruit juice (no sugar added), wine	Rinse with cold water, lay flat. Pour a capful of hydrogen peroxide onto stain and add a squirt of dish soap, rubbing it in with your finger in small circles. Rinse with cold water and repeat if necessary.	Make a borax or cornstarch paste and rub gently. *Avoid:* Vinegar.

TYPE OF STAIN	MY FAVORITE APPROACH	OTHER THINGS TO TRY
Sugar stains: ketchup, BBQ sauce, jellies, jams	Scrub gently with dish soap or laundry detergent in cold water, then rinse. Cup the stained portion of the fabric in your hand and pour (just-opened) club soda into your cupped hand. Swish the fizzing water around in your cupped hands, letting the bubbles fizz the stain loose. Repeat if necessary.	Soak in borax; sub hydrogen peroxide for club soda in my favorite approach. *Avoid*: Heat, liquid soap (glycerin will set sugar stains).
Ink, permanent marker	Lightly scrub with liquid soap, rinse, and then soak in rubbing alcohol.	*Avoid*: Heat.
Mold, mildew	Soak affected area in hydrogen peroxide.	Make a borax paste and scrub into stain.
Grass, rust	Soak stain in vinegar.	Rub gently with water and a few drops of Citra Solv, liquid soap (glycerin), or milk; or make a cream of tartar paste. *Avoid*: alkaline cleaners like baking soda and borax.

* Wherever I call for hydrogen peroxide, consider substituting a color-safe oxygen bleach like those offered from Seventh Generation, Ecover, or Biokleen. These contain hydrogen peroxide, but in a diluted concentration, so they won't discolor colored fabrics.

hand-wash how-to

My favorite method for tackling that little stack of hand-wash-only items mounting on the closet floor involves the bathroom sink and a tiny squirt of laundry detergent. The sink is usually the perfect size for containing most hand-washable items.

Step 1: Make sure sink is clean and free of toothpaste residue.

Step 2: Pull up the drain stopper (or use a drain plug), place the item in the sink, and begin filling with enough water to just cover the item. Your sink should never be more than half full, or else you'll splash water everywhere. Use the bathtub for large items.

Step 3: Add the tiniest amount of laundry detergent, as little as you can manage to pour (no more than a teaspoon).

Step 4: Create friction by repeatedly lifting the item up out of the water, smacking it down, and squeezing it out. You don't have to actually use a washboard, but think along those lines as you agitate the clothes. The more the item comes in contact with water and rubs up against itself, the more effective your detergent (aka dirt removal vehicle) will be. Your goal is to foster the contained use of force (key word: *contained*), not to agitate yourself by splashing water everywhere.

Step 5: Squeeze water and excess suds out of item gently. Drain the now-murky laundry detergent and water from the sink. Rinse item under cold water and squeeze more suds out.

141

Step 6: Fill sink once more with cold water, like you did in the beginning, and give the item a few more dunks in the fresh water to extract any lingering detergent residue.

Step 7: Squeeze as much water from the item as you can without wrenching and wringing it (you could damage gentler fabrics). Lay flat to dry on a wooden laundry drying rack or get hip to a clothesline.

clotheslines

Hanging your pretties out on the line is no longer reserved for the third-world chic. Five reasons why you might consider stringing one up:

1. You can hang rags when you're finished using them (so they don't mildew in the laundry pile).
2. Spare your door frames and shower bar by hanging your delicate, no-dryer items outside.
3. Sun drying (UV rays) kill germs and throw extra whitening power into the deal. (But be sure to hang bright colors on the line at night, so they don't fade in the sun.)
4. You save money on your gas or electricity bills by not running the dryer as often or as long.
5. It's fun to use clothespins in their intended capacity once in a while.

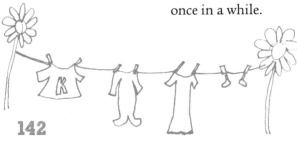

142

mending maven crash course

Anyone can perform basic mending. It's more a matter of getting into the spirit and getting yourself set up for success than of technical skill. As with all tasks described in this book, if you end up hating stitching and threadwork, then don't do it. Just know that you don't have to rely upon the dry cleaners for basic alterations and your favorite shirt isn't a lost cause when it loses a button.

tools of the trade

If your sewing kit is nonexistent (or in the back corner of the closet and hard to access), then you're probably not doing much with that stack of clothes in disrepair. Spruce up your kit, including the following mending and low-tech craft essentials:

- A good pair of scissors (that you only use on fabric and thread)
- A few spools of standard-colored thread (get colors that are likely to blend in with your basics, like black, white, and tan or cream)
- Needles (different sizes if you plan to use larger threads for decoration)
- Small stash of extra buttons
- Box of straight pins
- A few safety pins for holding things together between mending endeavors

Hip Trick

Keep mending essentials in a small bin or cute basket so you don't have to lug out a giant bin of sewing supplies, miscellaneous fabrics you didn't want to throw away, and hem tape from the early 1980s (you get the point) every time you need to repair something.

hip trick

Pulling a long set of threads through the length of your cloth can be really frustrating, especially when it forms a tangle on every stitch you make. Solve the tangling problem by dangling your needle below your fabric to let it spin itself free of twists. Don't double if you're stitching over a long distance (more than 18 inches, or the length from your fingers to your elbow).

If you're working on a longer project, I suggest meeting in the middle of whatever you're sewing with two doubled-up thread segments. I'm only good for about 24 inches of hand stitching in one sitting. Then I start to lose attention, get sloppy, and poke myself. No fun.

upgrades if you sew frequently

Things you'll want to add to your sewing kit as you start feeling fancy:

- ↳ Seam ripper
- ↳ A 2-inch see-through ruler, craft mat, and specialty sewing shears (which help you cut from above on a flat surface) for cutting fabric like a pro. A kit that includes all three usually runs about $45.

sewing vocabulary

Sewing reference books are particularly confusing, if you ask me. They assume you understand what the hell they're talking about, and the images are rarely helpful in the heat of the moment. The terms I've highlighted here are answers to my frustrations, common scenarios you might encounter in a bout with the mending pile. You generally don't need to know any of these terms. Most of them are commonsense things you can figure out (or just wing it) as you go. If you don't understand them, don't feel like your sewing future is doomed. Just take your new vocabulary (and a homemade treat) to a friend and ask for a visual demo.

what does it mean to double up thread?

Doubling up on thread is when you thread the needle and pull the tail so there are two equal lengths with which you will sew. Doubling your thread is an easy way to reinforce what you're stitching, but it can be a bummer since the threads can get tangled and knotted as you go along.

tying the knot

A no-vows-necessary approach to the most important step in any sewing project. Here are my favorite, tried-and-true methods for getting started (or finishing the job).

starting knot

If you're working with a single thread, wrap the thread around your finger three times, leaving a tail about an inch long. Carefully slip the stack of loops off your finger and tie the knot like usual, but sticking the tail through all three loops at once. Pull tight and voilà!

Are you using a doubled thread? My friend Liz showed me this fun trick for getting that initial knot in place:

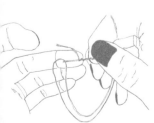

- ➥ Form a circle with the threaded needle, placing 2 inches of the tail on top of the needle and holding it down with your right thumb.
- ➥ Wind the tail over the top of the needle and back around (thread comes toward you), pressing your fingers firmly over the wound thread as you go so it doesn't unravel.

145

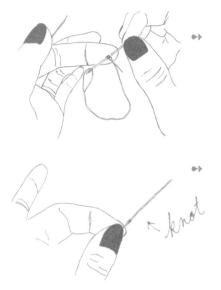
↝ knot

➥ Transfer your left index finger to the top of the needle in order to keep the wound thread from unraveling. Place your thumb on top of your index finger and then pull needle through with your right hand.

➥ As you pull, your left hand keeps a good grip on the wound section and you will feel it moving along the thread as you pull, ending up at the bottom of the thread and forming a sturdy knot. Tighten by pulling the tail. Voilà!

end knot

Slide your needle under a couple of stitches without pulling the thread all the way through. Stick your needle through the loop your thread forms and you've just made a knot. Repeat the process, attempting to grab the same group of stitches so your knots land on or near each other.

stitches that get the job done

All simple mending can be tackled with a few easy hand stitches. Though I vaguely recalled these from years of Girl Scout camp, a good friend's stepmom was able to clarify and beef up my vocabulary. (She teaches sewing classes, demystifying the needle and thread for people just like me all the time.)

Name your mending task; I have the hand stitch and how-to for you. Read on to find out how to tackle simple mending while you're catching up on podcasts after work.

146

mending holes and patchwork:
loop (whip) or running (straight) stitches

The loop or whip stitch wraps the thread around the cloth. This stitch is good for mending holes and sewing patches.

The running or straight stitch is when you go in one side and come out the other and then flip the thing over and repeat. This also works if you catch a few stitches and pull the thread through, a trick to speed things up. You just need to be sure you're catching no more than ¼-inch sections at a time or the thread paths on both sides of the fabric will end up looking like the dashed yellow lane markers on long stretches of highway.

finishing edges without a sewing machine:
blanket (buttonhole) stitch

Step 1: Start by poking your needle from the back of the fabric (if there is a front and a back; otherwise just designate one side as the back) to the front side and catching your knot on the fabric.

Step 2: Make your starting loop by guiding your needle over the top of the fabric and poking from the back of the fabric through to the front, but don't pull it tight; leave 1 inch of loop.

Step 3: Guide your needle through the loop, going right to left, and pull tight.

Step 4: Now you're ready to roll! Make a little U with

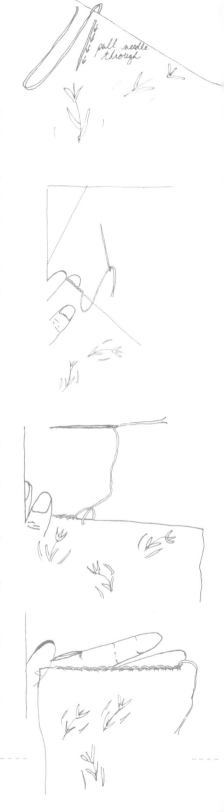

the base of your thread. Lead and grab the bottom of the U with your thumb.

Step 5: Poke your needle from the back of the fabric to the front side, making sure to come up ¼ inch (or less, depending on how far apart you want your stitches) to the right of your starting loop and that your thread U is on the left side of your needle.

Step 6: Pull through tightly and repeat.

Use regular thread to clean up a rough edge, or use thick craft thread (and a larger needle, minimum size 18) whenever you want to add a decorative finish to a plain edge (think a napkin or curtain edge).

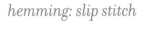

hemming: slip stitch

Step 1: Fold the fabric to desired length. (Do this by folding over twice, so you have a smooth fold at the point where you're stitching.) Pin or iron fabric to keep fold in place.

Step 2: You're going to sew from right to left, so insert the needle in the underside of the folded side pointing toward the left. Sticking it under the fold will hide it from view once you've finished hemming.

Step 3: Pick up a few threads (or a really tiny piece of fabric) from the non-folded side as close as possible to where the fold meets it. Don't pull the needle through just yet.

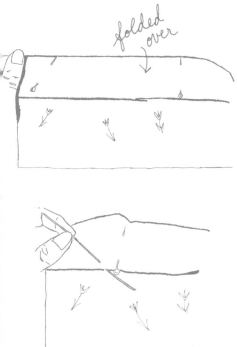

Step 4: Insert your needle immediately into the bottom of the fold. Run the needle along the inside of the fold and poke it out about ¼ inch to the left. Pull the thread all the way through.

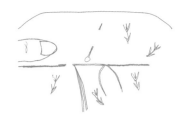

Step 5: Repeat grabbing small threads from the non-folded side just below where your needle exited the folded side.

Step 6: Admire your snazzy new hem!

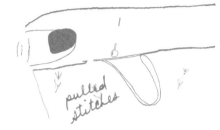

Hemming goes by pretty quickly because of the traveling you do with the needle inside the folded side. Plus, you can't really see the stitching on the reverse side since you've grabbed just a few threads.

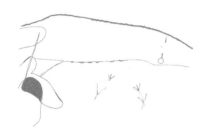

sewing a button

Reattaching a button (or swapping out a blah button with a wow button) takes about five minutes once you get the hang of it. It's a most impressive act of domesticity, up there with folding a fitted sheet (which you now know how to do because you read Chapter 3).

Step 1: Place a straight pin through the spot where you want your button to go. This just serves as a guide as you're getting your first couple stitches in place.

Step 2: Hide your knot underneath the button by sticking your needle into a spot right where you want your button

Word to the Wise

Stop stitching when you have only 2 inches remaining on your thread. Leave room for tying the end knot without going crazy.

needle-free sewing . . .

Fake it with a fun product called Stitch Witchery. Use it to finish an edge or hem without sewing. The tape bonds fabric when you iron it. If you mess up or change your mind down the road, all you need to do is reheat it and follow the directions on their website to remove the dried goo.

to go and grabbing a tiny (1/16-inch) piece of fabric.

Step 3: Pull your needle through the fabric and poke your needle through the underside of the button. The button should drop down onto the fabric and be facing the right direction, toward you.

Step 4: Position the button on the fabric and poke your needle through a diagonal hole (if the button has four holes) or the adjacent hole (if it has only two). This will mount your button, so make sure you insert the needle into the fabric in a location that's near where it will come out.

Step 5: Poke around the underside of the fabric to locate the first hole (where your first stitch came through the hole in the button) and loop through the same two holes a few times. Try to keep your stitches landing near previous ones so the reverse side isn't a mess of wild stitches.

Step 6: If your button has four holes, repeat for the other set of holes.

Step 7: Knot two or three times.

Note: If you're using a shank button (the kind with a hole or holes that are hidden and protruding from the underside of the button), you'll sew through its protrusion.

overwhelmingly easy craft projects

Have a go at one of these low-tech cloth craft projects on a rainy afternoon. I've managed to make them, so I can attest to their suitability for the especially uncoordinated (myself included).

lavender eye mask or
good-smelling sachets for your drawers

1. Cut out two small squares or rectangles from cute fabric (if you're making an eye mask, be sure you start with at least 8 inches of fabric).
2. Turn both squares inside out and use a running stitch on three of the four sides, ½ inch from the edge of the fabric.
3. Turn pouch right side out and fill it with desired contents (like dried lavender, dried citrus peels, and/or dry beans for weighting your eye mask).
4. Close fourth side by folding both edges inward inside the bag and finishing with a loop or slip stitch.

napkins

Cut up a colorful sheet that doesn't make a set any longer or has a stain, to make your own cloth napkins. Finish the edges with a decorative blanket stitch or invite yourself over to a friend's house to borrow her machine for the afternoon.

Hip Trick

Use your new end knot skills to tie a single knot every five or so stitches. If the hem ever gets caught and rips, it will only unravel in a small section instead of pulling out the whole thing.

pillows or pillow covers

1. Cut two same-size squares of fabric. With the right sides of the fabric together (so that the pillow covers will be inside out), use a running stitch along three sides of the squares (like with the eye mask/sachet project).
2. Stitch as much of the fourth side as you can, leaving room to either insert stuffing or squeeze the pillow inside once the fabric is turned right side out.
3. Finish with a loop or slip stitch.

strength in numbers

Assemble a few friends for periodic mending parties to get in the mood to mend. Ask pals to bring wine and snacks, and you provide a stash of needles and thread.

It was, in fact, at a mending party that I stopped fearing the machine, and now might consider getting my own at some point. Everyone doesn't need to own a sewing machine, though. Collective purchases and cooperative sewing gatherings are a great way to not eat the cost of tools and materials individually, plus you gain insight on how others tackle certain repair projects and you might even pick up new tricks. Try to find a few friends who are interested in going in on a little sewing club and you're in business (hopefully with at least one of you who knows how to operate the machine). Learn more about hosting a sewing party in Chapter 10.

resources

books

- *Better Basics for the Home: Simple Solutions for Less Toxic Living* by Annie Berthold-Bond.
  A nice resource for laundry and stain removal tips.
- *Cath Kidston's In Print* by Cath Kidston.
  I love this book because you don't actually have to know how to sew in order to incorporate many of her vintage cloth ideas and suggestions around the house.
- *The Complete Book of Sewing* by DK Publishing.
  Great pictures and step-by-step tutorials.
- *New Complete Guide to Sewing* by Reader's Digest.
  A good friend's favorite resource in her sewing library.
- *Sew U: The Built by Wendy Guide to Making Your Own Wardrobe* by Wendy Mullen.
  Another great resource for beginning sewers.

web

- Jo-Ann Fabric and Craft Stores (joann.com). Frequent sales on fabrics and good deals on sewing supplies.
- Colette Patterns (colettepatterns.com). Crafty projects, how-tos, and an inspiring blog to help you get started.
- Burda Style (burdastyle.com). Tips, techniques, learning resources, and fancy project ideas.

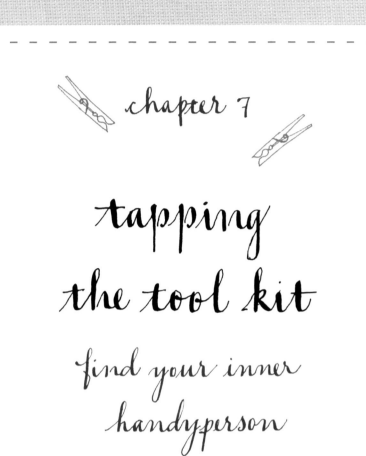

chapter 7

tapping the tool kit

find your inner handyperson

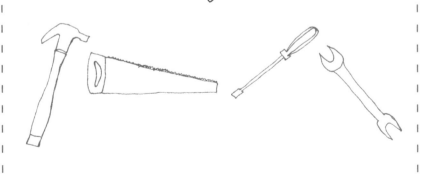

The less time you spend stressing out over how to handle quick-fix things around the house, the more time you can spend doing things you like. This chapter is geared at encouraging creative problem solving, helping you to conjure up your inner Girl or Boy Scout.

First we'll cover all the tools a happy home homie should have lying around, and then we'll get into setting yourself up for improvisation success. When you start to solve home problems with a stash of things like bungee cords, dowels, and binder clips, you get to reallocate time spent wandering through hardware stores and money spent paying people to fix stuff for you.

It's empowering to fix something yourself, no matter how simple. I tend to quickly fix things for functionality and then address the fix later if my impromptu crafty solution bugs me. Making do until you can get to the hardware store or find the right deal on whatever materials you need is an art in itself. I haven't yet found a good fold-up table, one I can use for yard sales or crafts, for free on the side of the road, so I'll continue to rig up my table extension, which you'll read about later in the chapter.

A few years ago my dad took me to the hardware store, where we selected a table saw as my birthday present. I'd been itching for one ever since I went to a carpenter friend's woodworking shop and cut up cute art blocks out of one of the boards that made up my former cinder-block-and-board bookcase. I never did take that table saw out of the box, but I'm not ashamed to

Word to the Wise

You get what you pay for in the tool aisle. Select a midrange tool over bottom-of-the-line options. It's better to pay a little more for one tool than to have to buy a second when the first one breaks or doesn't work properly.

admit it. Eventually I sold it on Craigslist and used the money on what I get more use out of on a daily basis: groceries.

As with all subjects covered in this book, home handiwork skills include a knowledge of the bare-bones basics and ways to be fancier about the work if you so choose. Using a table saw is certainly on the fancier end of the skill spectrum. I hope that after reading this chapter you'll identify unique solutions and implement your own creative ideas that pertain to your home situation.

This chapter does come with a minor disclaimer: please weigh the costs when considering fixing something yourself. If it's possible to break it even further, how much does a new one cost? Knowing when to call someone who knows what he or she is doing is key, even if that person is just a pal who's had a similar problem.

taking stock

Let's have a look at what's in your tool kit. These are the basic tools any household should stock. You don't want to be at home without them.

- One Phillips-head and one flat-head screwdriver (you don't really need the big, fancy screwdriver kit)
- Mini screwdriver kit, for tiny things (like eyeglass and iPhone screws)
- Hammer
- Hardware kit (or an assortment of screws, nails, and anchors)
- Wire cutter
- Adjustable wrench
- Pliers

upgrade ideas from readers

I asked my blog readers about their favorite tools. Here are three great suggestions for fancying up your tool kit (or adding to your wish list):

1. Dremel tools do all sorts of handy things like cutting (metal, wood, and tile), sanding, and routing

2. A hex key is that little L-shaped thing you get in every IKEA tool baggie. A set of hex keys can help you open up just about anything you have around the house.

3. Stud finder. This device detects studs (ideal places to hang heavy things on the wall) and also scans for metal and wires (not ideal places to sink a nail).

- Tape measure
- Small handsaw
- 9-inch torpedo level for hanging pictures and other small household tasks
- Sharpening stone and oil for maintaining household scissors, knife blades, and other tools
- Five-in-one tool (a painter's tool that can be used for spackle and nail removals)

where to stash your tools

Most basic toolboxes have one big compartment and a little tray on top, which can lead to an unorganized and jumbled tool and hardware mess. My mom has always sworn by the fishing supply aisle, and not because she's into bait and tackle. A tackle box has more slots and ways to segregate hardware than a box specially made for tools, plus tackle boxes are usually cheaper.

If you don't have a utility room, don't keep your tools under the kitchen sink. You don't want to have to dig around under there every time you need to fix or hang something, and they might get water damage. We keep our tools in our all-purpose everything closet.

Other cool tool-stashing ideas I've seen:

- Back-of-door hanging shoe rack with clear pockets

⟶ Long pieces of leather or canvas nailed to a board (which in turn is attached to a wall) with loops between the nails to hang tools

drill skills

The only power tool you really need to own (or share with a friend) is a power drill. You can find a decent one for about $50. I recommend a corded drill for the following reasons:

⟶ It will be lighter than a cordless drill (no monster-sized battery to lug around).
⟶ Corded drills are generally more powerful and you don't have to worry about whether or not the battery is charged when you want to use it.
⟶ A cordless drill's battery life expectancy goes down the less you use it (and the longer you own it), so the occasional user will get less bang for the buck by going with a cordless.

The trickiest part of using a power drill is holding it steady and knowing when you've reached the right tension with the screw, so as not to strip it. You don't have to use force (as you would with a screwdriver), but you have to have a firm grasp and an intentional attitude.

Drill tips:

⟶ Predrilling (or piloting) a hole with a bit that's narrower than your screw is pretty helpful in most drill jobs. Be sure the hole is smaller than the base of the

159

screw (not just the external thread) or it will be too big and your screw will end up pulling out.

- ⬦ You can buy a set of drill bits and then proceed to drill any size hole into nearly anything you can imagine, like transforming an ordinary 5-gallon bucket into a fancy planter by drilling drainage holes.

- ⬦ If possible, get a drill with two handles (one on the base and another near the drill head). This gives you a better vantage and allows you to apply a more even grip. I love using my Craftsman drill with its (removable) second handle.

anchor basics

Anchors are great for hanging things on walls and ceilings where there is no convenient wood stud or beam behind the surface. An anchor's stability depends on a couple of factors: direction of pull and surrounding material composition.

You need a *threaded drywall anchor* if your wall/ceiling is thin (a nail or screw goes right in and you can pull it out easily). Choose metal for a few cents more than the plastic. You can drill or screw it directly into the wall.

Pick up a metal *toggle bolt* or a *collapsing metal sleeve anchor* (sometimes called a molly bolt) to secure heavy objects. Be sure to get metal. The cheapie plastic expansion anchors always bend and warp (and drive me batty) as I'm trying to hammer them into the predrilled hole. Both of these kinds of anchors will require you to predrill a hole as wide as the anchor.

Never use a plastic expansion anchor for hanging things from the ceiling.

move-in/move-out skills

You want your deposit back in full? Patch the nail holes, people. It seems like this simple feat is all too often ignored in the turnover of rental properties. It's no fun to arrive in a new-to-you home and find a bunch of nails that used to hold up other people's stuff.

Go through the house with your claw hammer (the kind of hammer that has a curved tail on the head) and pull out the hardware road map of your (or the previous tenant's) décor. Just unscrew anchored hardware, as in most cases anchors themselves are not easily removable.

Spackle paste comes in pint-sized buckets and often in squeeze tubes. I prefer the squeeze tube because it has a better chance of not drying out between uses. Squeeze or apply spackle paste into holes, then flatten and smooth the surface with a putty knife, five-in-one tool, or even the edge of a ruler. Let dry, and you're done. Easy breezy.

You'll want to sand the completely dry spackled patches with a medium-grit sandpaper to even out the surface if you're also repainting.

installing shelving and hanging pictures

It only takes a few extra moments to grab a level and a pencil and make a few marks to be sure your wall hangings are straight. Your perfectionist efforts will pay off when you don't have to reinstall the shelf or add another anchor ½ inch higher than the original one because staring at crooked shelves or slanted pictures every day started to drive you nuts.

Hip Trick
Install an anchor and then screw in a vintage or quirky drawer pull to be used as a knob to hang pictures, necklaces, or other objects by using a lightweight wire.

161

The best way to hang large pictures and other heavy objects is to use two anchors (and two screws) when possible.

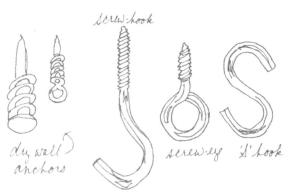

screw-hook

dry wall anchors

screw-eye   'S' hook

creative ways to hang things from the ceiling

Screw hooks are my favorite way to suspend lights, vegetable baskets, and bamboo room dividers from the ceiling.

In most cases you'll be fine screwing the hook directly into the ceiling without an anchor and hanging your object. If your object is corded (i.e., a light), secure the dangling cord with a nail or two along the wall or corner to keep the cord away from the light and allow it to hang properly. You'll know if you need an anchor if you give the screw hook a gentle tug and it pulls right out.

Follow directions for weight limits listed on the screw hook's package (or by talking to someone at the hardware store if they're sold loose). Generally, a standard screw hook holds up to 40 pounds, so you should be fine. Look specifically for a ceiling hook kit if you'd like to hang chandeliers, plants, or other heavy objects. The kit's package will indicate maximum load.

Sometimes ceilings are just downright crappy and can't support anything. You can still hang your wire vegetable basket in the kitchen from a single curtain rod support. You just need to be sure to get a bracket that juts out far enough from the wall to allow the basket to hang properly (not skewed at a dangerous angle so your potatoes threaten to pelt passersby).

hip and handy

Handy home fixery is based on two principles: curiosity and observation. Ever since I was a kid, my favorite method for discovery and innovation has been to carefully dissemble the item in question and see what's going on in there. That's not always practical or possible, so creative improvisation around the house goes more smoothly with a good stash of supplies to work with.

This is my quintessential list of handy things to have around the house at all times:

- ➼ *Bungee cords* (at least three long and three short).
- ➼ *Twine.* You'll encounter a few different kinds in the rope and binding aisle. Look for the stiffer and extremely sturdy *sisal twine* for tough outdoor projects, and be sure to get the softer *jute twine* for easy twisting and tying, great for both indoor and outdoor use.
- ➼ *Wire.* Look for 22- to 28-gauge galvanized steel wire; it's totally bendable and wire cutters snip it easily. The list of things you can do in the hanging realm with this wire is endless. Wire has helped me hang four picture frames in a row

Hip Trick

Hang unframed artwork or paintings with four medium-sized nails. Hammer in the nails (leaving about ½ inch out), two in the bottom and two around the top. Holding the piece (to keep it from falling on top of you), carefully hammer the bottom nails upward and in toward the artwork. Repeat for the top nails. Don't smash them into the painting. Tilting them inward is usually enough to hold the piece securely on the wall.

hip trick

Get ideas for crafty solutions by paying attention to how others maximize small spaces. Restaurant and store bathrooms in big cities are my fave place to pick up nifty tricks for DIY shelving and storage. They are often the smallest rooms you'll find anywhere, and shopkeepers must get creative with stashing cleaning and supply stocks.

Art galleries are also great places to pay attention to (and steal) creative installation ideas for your own wall hangings.

using only two nails, display my prized windowpanes from our boring chain-link backyard fence, and suspend a strawberry jar from my neighbor's back deck.

- *Spare plywood sheet* (sturdy, flat, clean wood). Ideally you'd find something on the side of the road, but buying a 4-by-8-foot piece of plywood at the hardware store is not going to break the bank. The sheet will run you about $20. Have the handy folks at the hardware store cut it down for you while you're there; a 4-by-6-foot size is ideal for all your table extend-ing purposes. If you can transport it and have a place to stash it, you could even keep the whole sheet intact. You don't need anything fancy; C-grade plywood or sheathing board will do.
- *Indoor extension cords.* Try to find ones with three-pronged receptacles so that you can plug in any type of electronic device.
- *Utility clamps.* We already covered the usefulness of clothespins in Chapter 1, so having a couple of giant, super-strong versions of a clothespin lying around makes life even better.

- **Zip ties.** Use these little plastic cinching cords to affix just about any two objects. I've used them to secure milk crates to my bicycle rack and hang a box fan from the ceiling using two screw eye hooks.

- **Binder clips.** In case you slept through Photo Hanging 101, binder clips are a fun way to display an unframed photo on the wall without poking holes in it with a nail or pin. Clamp your paper (or other lightweight object) and hang one of the loop handles from a nail or push pin. Office supply stores sell binder clips that are a notch above the standard black ones. Deck your walls with all silver clips or other fun colors until you have time to figure out framing.

- **Dowels.** I love these wooden rods almost as much as I love clothespins. They're cheap, they're handy to have around the house, and they can double as curtain rods (suspended from binder clips) in a pinch.

Wooden
↖ dowels

You can formulate all sorts of home solutions and creative improvisations with a fully stocked utility closet. It's time to start taking theory into practice, my hip friends. The next time you're faced with going to the hardware, home, or garden supply store, think about the simple mechanics of your ideal solution. Sure, there's something you could go out and buy, but could you also make it just as easily?

Go to your tool and utility space and see if you have anything that might work in lieu of what they're selling. Here are a few project ideas to inspire a new outlook in using things you already have.

extending your tabletop space

Hosting dinner parties, potlucks, and craft gatherings really ends up boiling down to table space (as you'll see in Chapter 10). If you own a fold-up 4-by-8-foot yard sale or craft table or by some chance landed a grown-up dinner table with actual extenders, then ignore this project idea. For all the rest of us out there who are tabletop (and potentially counter space) challenged, don't worry, you're not doomed to entertain on the floor.

You might not be very surprised to find out that my MO for special home-based events is to beg, borrow, or visit the thrift store. We even found a decent table on the side of the road. It's a square card table, pseudo-sturdy, slightly shorter and fatter than our existing square dinner table.

Here's where being handy and taking a few moments to slow down and improvise comes in. Both my kitchen table and the found card table are 3 feet square. The first time I combined them (the afternoon before a dinner gathering) I realized that what I had in mind—placing a large wooden plank across the tops of both to make one large table—was a no-go, because the wood was warped from summer humidity.

We also had a smaller, square plywood board, slightly shorter than the two tables' width, and it had two small holes about the size of quarters drilled into opposite sides. I whipped out various bungee cords and hooked them through the holes in the plywood (in

THE HIP GIRL'S GUIDE TO HOMEMAKING

case of animated dinner conversations) and shoved books along the perimeter of a second wood plank stuck in for extra stability (and to help level out the 1½-inch slope from kitchen table to card table), making a flat surface for guests. I topped the whole affair with a vinyl craft tablecloth to buffer the books against spills.

Later that evening, guests were none the wiser that below the cups, plates and my great grandma's lace tablecloth lurked layers of improvisation.

building a trellis or tomato plant cage

This simple and particularly magical combination of dowels and twine will save you money at the garden store and leave you with reusable materials to construct another specialized structure as your garden and outdoor space needs change.

Supplies needed:

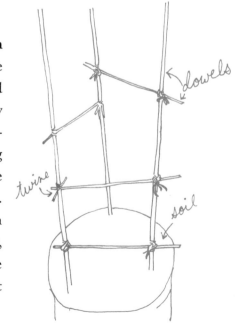

•▸ **Two to four ½-inch-diameter wooden dowels** (or wood molding pieces) for the base. Taking into consideration what kind of structure you're going to make and how high you need it to go, you can find the longer pieces of wood molding in the flooring section of the hardware store. They come in quarter-rounds and rectangular shapes. When building a cage for vines and bean plants, the molding pieces are the tallest, sturdiest, and cheapest materials for the job; dowels (48 inches long) work great for bushy plants like tomatoes that need support most at the base. (My cucumbers have topped their 8-foot cage supports, so I'm glad I gave them enough room!)

- ↦ **Two 1/8-inch-diameter dowels** cut into three or four pieces to serve as ledges between the legs of the base. Cut them to fit the distance between the legs.
- ↦ **Jute twine** cut into 12-inch pieces; start with ten pieces and cut more if you need them.

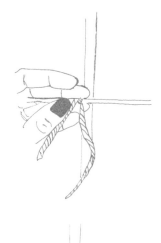

Step 1: Insert the ½-inch dowels in the ground (or in containers if you have 'em) to form the base structure of your trellis or cage.

Step 2: Wrap twine around a small dowel to form a couple of loops. Leave a 3-inch tail.

Step 3: Tightly wrap the long end of the twine around the top of the base to anchor the small dowel to the base. Continue wrapping twine around the small dowel where it meets the base. Continue until you have just enough of a tail to meet the original 3-inch tail. There's no right way to do this; just be sure you're keeping the twine tight. You don't want there to be any slack between the layers of twine or else your dowel will come loose.

Step 4: Tie the two tails together, knot twice, and repeat on the other end to form a ledge connecting two of the base legs. Make as many ledges as you need.

168

You can also use this method to add a ledge to an existing deck railing for plants to climb and rest on, which maximizes the utility of your existing structure.

share your toys

Another good reason to get to know your neighbors (beyond sharing food and fun) might be to form a tool-share collective. It's pretty silly for people who live near each other to all own the same power tools. A tool-share group can be as organized as you care to make it, which means you and the upstairs neighbor might occasionally swap power tools to complete home projects or the guy across the street uses his free-standing garage to house your street's collective stash of tools, which might be checked out on an as-needed basis.

There are considerations that should be discussed in advance, like how your group handles responsibility for broken items or what rules surround borrowing from the group.

resources

books

- ↠ *The Sharing Solution: How to Save Money, Simplify Your Life & Build Community* by Janelle Orsi and Emily Doskow. *Great primer on how to start a tool-share (and all other types of sharing groups) with friends, neighbors, or local community members.*

169

- *Dare to Repair: A Do-It-Herself Guide to Fixing (Almost) Anything in the Home* by Julie Sussman and Stephanie Glakas-Tenet.

web

- Ace Hardware (acehardware.com). Step-by-step how-to and FAQ sections online. In-store customer assistance is also top-notch, and there are Ace stores across the country.
- The Natural Handyman (naturalhandyman.com). A wealth of information about home repair things most of us know little about. The handyman writer is quirky and explains hardware and construction recommendations well.

Part III

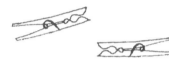

Life After

Restaurants

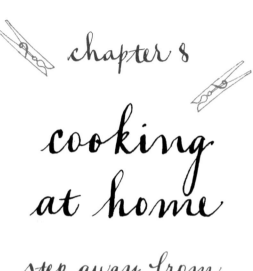

chapter 8

cooking at home

step away from the takeout menu

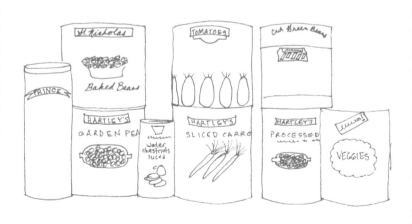

Let's be reasonable: a single chapter won't do the kitchen justice. However, a new attitude and a few baby steps in the direction of cooking and eating at home will set you on an exciting new track to not hating (or fearing) your kitchen.

First, I need to share a few things I'm probably not supposed to tell you: I don't enjoy the everyday aspect of cooking, and you'll never hear me say how therapeutic it is to put dinner together every night (though, pounding the hell out of a dough ball is cathartic—see the bread making section). I'm the special projects coordinator of our house, i.e., good at flashy, every few days kinds of things, not everyday things. I'm not great at following directions and I pride myself on imprecision (yes, gasp, even as our house's baker and pastry maker).

I don't read newspaper and magazine articles on gourmet food. I don't like it when people use the word *phenomenal* in reference to food (or ever, really). I wouldn't consider myself a foodie, and I'm still shocked when people refer to me as a food blogger/writer. If I can learn to love the kitchen under these circumstances, then certainly you can too.

In this chapter, we'll start with the basics, like how to grocery-shop. We'll move on to building your kitchen ecosystem, inserting homemade items gradually, then phase into a functioning, pride-inducing kitchen that's ready for anything, like making dinner.

Open your fridge right now. Can you make a meal with anything in there at this very moment? Let's change what you have on hand from sriracha sauce, a couple of containers of yogurt, and a rock-hard lemon into ready-to-use components of meals. In the next chapter we'll cover how to stash meal components (in the freezer or in jars on the back shelf of your pantry) so they don't go bad before you get to them.

Developing a relationship with your kitchen is less about touting easy and fast ways to be an at-home gourmet (which are handy tips to seek) and more about actually using your kitchen as a grown-up. This means taking charge of what goes into your body (something restaurant eating frequently prohibits) and how great it feels when the tide miraculously shifts and it eventually becomes more convenient to cook at home than eat out.

food stamped

My first year in New York City went pretty much just how I expected: a slideshow of random odd jobs (dog walking, kid schlepping, paid research studies), working for grizzly editors demanding rewrites (this does not include my wonderful book editor, Julia!), and enough bustling to warrant weekly teary breakdowns.

I didn't, however, anticipate living way below the poverty level. My girlfriend was a full-time student (at a school we couldn't afford), and my odd jobs barely kept my half of the rent, my own student loans, and our phone bill paid.

We applied for food stamps after a student friend of ours said we'd probably qualify. My girlfriend passed in our qualifying interview with flying colors, though she still had to show that she had a part-time job (which she did). My situation was a little trickier—I had to provide letters from the people I was freelancing for that showed a rate and number of hours per week or month. I lied and told my "clients" that I needed said letters for tax purposes (because who wants to hire a freelancer who's on food stamps?).

We were able to do it right and apply as a household, since

that's what we are: two adults who share a fridge and three meals a day. We received a little blue credit card with my girl-friend's picture on it and a new acronym, EBT (electronic benefit transfer). Each month $201 would appear in our online balance.

grocery store game change

As a single lass, the only relationship I'd ever shared with grocery shopping involved luxuriously selecting recipes (that involved a bunch of stuff I didn't have in the cabinets), overbuying out of grocery store excitement, and then pitching out the decaying and compost-ready food two weeks later. When I moved to New York—and into cohabitation 2.0, grown-up edition—I no longer had the luxury of that kind of waste. (Nor should anyone, really, but that's another story.)

With a budget of $201 to spend for an entire month's worth of food for two people, I began to understand why my previous method wasn't working. Like with a smart wardrobe, we needed interchangeable components in our food system.

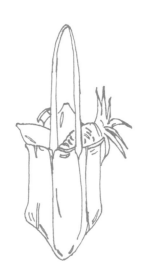

ditch the recipe

Single-recipe shopping and cooking is expensive and unreasonable (unless you're going to make that recipe every single week, as may be the case for bread or other staple recipes). Think of your dinner plate as a Trivial Pursuit game piece and break it down into components. There are three main categories that should populate your cart: greens, grains, and proteins. Here's a list of what we regularly stock in our kitchen.

fruits and veggies

Usually two or three vegetable options for the week:

Collard greens	Swiss chard
Dandelion greens	Kale
Spinach	Broccoli

snackable fruits and veggies

Carrots: buy the whole ones and cut them up yourself, it saves money and energy (carrots don't grow in the snack-shape you'll see bagged in the store)

Apples, oranges, or other fruits you can toss in your purse or bag when you're on the go

Sugar snap peas: these are one of my fave snacky foods

While in the produce area of the store, don't forget to grab a few staples, such as onions and garlic, and maybe carrots, tomatoes, or other veggies that you'll use the week you buy them.

grains

We keep grains on hand in quart-sized mason jars, which help keep them fresh by sealing out our pantry air. We keep stashes of:

Quinoa	Amaranth
Brown rice	Corn (for stovetop popping)
Arborio rice	Buckwheat
(the rice for risotto)	

Non-gluten-free households might also include in their grains stash:

Couscous   *Farro*

Barley   *Bulgur*

proteins

I won't get too high-school-nutrition-class on you here, but the healthiest diet includes various sources of protein, including lean animal proteins and hearty vegetable/grain protein complements.

Here are some ideas to get you started on diversifying your protein intake:

Beans

Tempeh

Tofu

Pastured and sustainably raised meats. (Read on in the chapter if you're grumbling about how expensive these can be. Good meat should really be considered a special occasion supplement to a steady base of non-animal sources of protein.)

Fish, especially sardines or anchovies. I've learned to like them because small fish are an affordable source of omegas (best kind of fat you can get) and contain the lowest amounts of mercury contamination. Generally speaking, the larger the fish, the higher up on the food chain you're going thus the more exposure to contaminants you're getting.

food in a box?

We all have our own food preferences, and many of us have dietary restrictions. You may be vegetarian, vegan, lactose intolerant, allergic to nuts, sensitive to alcohol or carbs or sugar . . . the list goes on and on. In our house, we're gluten free. For us, this ingredient omission cuts out most of the packaged, heavily processed things out there trying to pass as food.

Regardless of your diet, when you're on a really tight budget, packaged foods are usually the first thing to go anyway, but you don't have to be gluten free to understand why a super-long ingredients list is not good for your body. Packaged foods are generally made to endure long shelf lives (even the organic and better-ingredient versions), which means they're often chock-full of chemicals your body can't process. For a thorough description, I'll defer here to Michael Pollan's *Food Rules*, one of them being: if a third-grader can't pronounce it, you probably shouldn't be eating it.

When you attempt to make things at home, you don't need all the additives and preservatives because you're just going to eat it, not wrap it in plastic and drive it around the country for a month.

putting the pieces together

We shop to set ourselves up for success with interchangeable proteins and greens, simple stir-fry dishes, risotto combinations, and basic meat-and-potatoes kinds of meals.

Word to the Wise

Don't get grocery greedy. Remember, you can come back to the store next week (or tomorrow). You're not stocking up for a nuclear fallout, or at least not yet. Check out Chapter 9 for details on a small-batch lifestyle.

179

We buy eggs, milk, olive oil, almond milk, raisins, nuts, coffee, spices, flour, and chocolate bars (of course) on an as-needed basis. The key to all this is planning. We make lists before going to the store, building upon what is already in the house. With the three-component system, the meal options start popping out, and the produce that's being used up trumps (or shapes) our gastronomic whims.

Start using your fridge more as the source for what you eat each day, rather than as that big white thing collecting crumbs, grime, and rotting food (an expensive compost pile).

Food stamps taught us that we can eat well (non-GMO, mostly organics, and a lot of local or farmers' market items) for no more than $250 a month. Let's do some math: that's roughly $8.33 per day for two adults. Two people can eat from home all month for what it costs to buy two mediocre lattes every day. We no longer need food stamps, but we still spend less than $300 per month on three meals a day from home, and we eat so well. Changing how we shopped was key, but here are a few places that help us (and others) keep grocery costs low.

- **Food co-ops.** Most cities have food cooperatives in addition to regular grocery stores, and these co-ops all work a little differently in terms of benefits and requirements for membership. They often involve an initial membership fee or option to work a regular volunteer shift for reduced prices. Retail grocery prices are double, sometimes triple what stores pay. If you can join a cooperative that cuts out some of these costs in any way, do it!

- **Buying clubs.** Round up a small group of friends or households to go in together on large orders—meats, vegetables, basic groceries, or hard-to-find things like canning supplies. You'll essentially be forming your own mini co-op. Organizing and coordinating the logistics of large orders may be a learning curve at first, but when you and twenty friends (or five or six households) start saving a bunch of money, you won't be complaining. You'll also learn a lot about local and regional farms, companies you want to support, and what are the best deals to be had.

- **Rebranded products.** Places like Trader Joe's, Aldi, Whole Foods Market, and oftentimes your local grocer rebrand products purchased from brand-name companies. Ever wonder how they can offer the low prices they tout? These stores will either make large cash purchases (a huge incentive for producers) or just exercise buying power on overstock items that companies inevitably end up producing.

    The downside to all this money-saving commotion is that you don't really know what company made whatever it is you're buying, and you (being hip to all this) know that it's good to know as much as possible about the things you're buying and consuming. What you do know is that an individual store's ethics dictate what companies/distributors it purchases from, so if you're shopping this way, be sure you understand what your store supports. I prefer shopping for olive oil, paper products, and other higher-ticket monthly items at Whole Foods under their 365 Everyday Value brand. I understand their company policy and ethics, plus, they occasionally have overstock (and thus good prices on) humanely raised meats.

- ↦ **CSAs—community-supported agriculture.** CSAs are available everywhere and in all sorts of forms. How it works: you "buy in" to a farm with a one-time annual payment (half or whole shares cost an average of $200 or $500, respectively) and each week during the growing season you get a box full of locally produced fruit and veggies grown on your farm. Ours works out to about $26 per week for a full-share (a huge bounty) of fruits and vegetables.

- ↦ **Farmers' market deals.** Contrary to popular belief, the farmers' market is not boutique shopping. (Do you really think you're getting the better end of the bargain for apples—or anything—that have been doused in pesticides and have traveled more than 2,000 miles to get to you?) Aside from the fact that small farmers make most of their income from direct sales at the market, market prices are usually comparable to what you'll see at a Whole Foods or supermarket where you'd actually want to eat the produce. And farmers' markets are hot spots for finding natural, local produce. You, the discerning, hip individual that you are, understand

Word to the Wise

CSAs can be an overwhelming commitment for someone not accustomed to cooking at home at least four meals a week. Even a half share will be a drastic influx of fresh produce, a ticking bomb of composting grocery anxiety. Go in on it with a committed (and, better yet, experienced) friend or roommate.

that image isn't everything and that fruits or veggies that aren't magazine-cover-worthy are not to be dismissed.

As the season is wrapping up, farmers like to unload as much of their harvest as possible. (They want to go on vacation, if they're lucky.) As you start to tune into what's in season—by going to the market every weekend—you'll notice when harvest abundance flags clearance prices. Also noteworthy: farmers' "seconds" are perfectly acceptable. My grandma grew up foraging behind supermarkets for seconds during the Depression. Farmers bring their seconds to the market but usually keep them stashed away; ask any vendor if he or she has seconds for a lower price. Slice off the bruise and dig in.

➻ **Shop around.** Frugal shoppers know not only where to buy the things they need but also average price ranges for those items. You really should know what the things you buy regularly cost, and hence when a great deal is looking you in the face. Sure, this method requires trips to a few different places and actually paying attention to what you buy, but in the end it's really worth it when you've saved $20 a month for a whole year. Savings add up faster than you'd expect, especially when you're pinching pennies in the first place.

Hip Trick

Spend a few dollars on reusable cloth bags to use for grains and bulk purchases and you'll cut packaging out of the picture entirely. These bags can usually be found near a store's bulk section or check online.

There are endless creative solutions to eating well on a budget, but they involve a little more foresight, and in some cases a little extra legwork. Can you dig it, or does that bland deli-bought sandwich really make your day?

bulk binge

Hit up your grocery store's bulk bin section; if your store doesn't have one, start shopping elsewhere. Paying by the pound for as much (or as little) as you need is the most cost-effective way to shop. Moreover, why pay someone to put something in a container that's probably bad for the planet, anyway? Best buys in the bulk section include sugars, flours, nuts, and dry beans. And let's not forget spices. Buying those artfully prepackaged spice containers is like stuffing money into a container of the same size and sending it off to sea. Buy small quantities of the spices called for in a recipe and stop throwing away half a container's worth of year-old spices.

reduce your convenience consumption

Pay premiums for things like organic produce, *not* for easy-to-do-yourself convenience items. Stop buying:

- **Flavored yogurts.** Plain yogurt is a perfect medium for whatever flavor you're in the mood for. Adding a touch of maple syrup, vanilla extract, or blueberry jam (really, whatever you have on hand) is the most cost- and mood-effective way to always have a variety of flavors at your disposal.

184

- **Precut sticks of butter.** Oil is usually a healthier option, but if you're going to use butter, go for the glory here, the 32-ouncer. Surely you have a cutting board and a sharp knife. Why would you opt for someone to cut it for you? Precision is overrated; you'll figure out how to make the pieces even enough after a few tries. I pay half the price of four sticks of pre-cut butter for the same quantity of French (translate: amazing) butter. Plus if you're going to try clarifying butter, which I recommend, you should not buy precut sticks for this fun little chore. You'd be wasting your time and money.

- **Salad dressing.** A basic vinaigrette is the simplest thing to make out of things I know you already have in the fridge and pantry. There are a ton of ways to be fancier about it, of course, but a spot of olive oil, rice or wine vinegar, salt, and pepper will give you a non-preservative-laden option for your greens.

- **Precut vegetables.** Come on! If you're too busy to slice up a zucchini, we gotta talk. This is most likely not even an issue because pre-cut veggies usually come on a Styrofoam tray with cling wrap, and you've boycotted Styrofoam (right?) because it never biodegrades. You may also be buying bagged or canned precut veggies. If so, listen up, take notes, put a Post-it on your forehead. When it comes to quantities, simple experience shows us that it's cheaper when you buy more. No, you don't have to go to Costco, just begin to take note of types of convenience you're

Hip Trick

Do yourself a favor and buy the quart of yogurt and a set of small glass Tupperware containers. You'll save money (and possibly the planet) while you're at it.

COOKING AT HOME

consuming, especially when buying individually packaged things. How much longer does it really take to put a few spoonfuls of yogurt in a Tupperware container?

the grocery shopper's dilemma

These are the two most basic things to keep in mind at the grocery store: understanding local and organic and why you should incorporate both into your diet. I'm not coming from the position or ideology of luxury here. We take our food (and what it ate before we eat it) very seriously.

- **Local.** Since you've started your garden (Chapter 4, wink, wink) you're getting hip to what's in season in your area. Moreover, you've tasted lettuce or tomatoes you grew yourself, consuming your backyard or stoop harvest just minutes after plucking it from the ground or vine; you're starting to see what things are *really* supposed to taste like.

  Beyond taste, buying locally grown foods is important in reestablishing regional food systems, which strengthen local economies, cut down on travel/pollution costs and provide communities with nutrient-dense, fresh foods.

  Seasonal and local are not always synonymous; for example, citrus is seasonal during winter months in the United States, yet only a handful of US states are suitable for growing citrus. Giving up lemons, limes, and oranges because you live in New York is a little extreme. It's okay to buy Florida oranges, just know they're in season when weather cools off and try to eat local ones then.

Buy what you can locally and make a point of sourcing things that don't grow in your area during appropriate seasons for your surrounding regions. Hint: if it's coming all the way from South America or Spain, it's most likely not supposed to be in season when you're eating it.

↠ **Organic.** We try to buy mostly organic or minimally treated foods, and belonging to a food co-op helps make this affordable for us. Sadly, not everyone has that kind of option. For supermarket shoppers, meats and milk are an organic must. Industrial meat producers' feedlot practices are enough to send you permanently to the tofu aisle. By choosing organic, you're basically paying more money for what's not included in your dinner: pesticides, synthetic fertilizers, genetic modifications, antibiotics, and growth hormones. But if you choose to eat meat, it's well worth it.

The "organic" label, like all large-scale regulatory things, is imperfect at times. Knowing as much as possible about the company touting an organic label (or about the regional farms who can't swing organic designation because of either financial or practical obstacles) is your

buy unsalted butter!

- Baking and cooking often require unsalted butter because you add specific amounts of salt or salty items with other foods and don't need extra in your butter.
- You get to choose the quality and quantity of salt when you add it. I'll sprinkle a dash of sea salt on a piece of buttered toast for the salted butter effect, and I know I'm eating top-quality sodium.

187

best bet. Marketing is slick, so cut through the fat by talking with friends and grocery store staff and checking the good ol' interwebs.

Here's a short list to jot down and toss into your wallet: which produce you should always buy organic, and when supplementing with conventionally grown fruits and veggies is okay. If you're buying conventional produce, try to select a locally produced option (or at least something from your own time zone).

Must Buy Organic	Conventionally Grown Okay
Apples	*Bananas*
Cherries	*Blueberries*
Strawberries	*Oranges, tangerines*
Peaches	*Avocadoes*
Pears	*Broccoli*
Grapes (imported)	*Cabbage*
Leafy greens, like lettuce, kale, Swiss chard, and spinach	*Radishes*
	Onions
	Sweet potatoes
Peppers	
Celery	

Visit these online resources before you shop to further develop your grocery store glossary:

→ Eat Well Guide (eatwellguide.org), to figure out what's local, in season, and sustainably produced in your area.
→ Animal Welfare Approved (animalwelfareapproved

.org/consumers/food-labels), to make sense of all the different things labels will say at the store, plus understand some limitations of labeling.

throes of cooking (so you don't throw in the towel)

Now, don't panic if you haven't set foot in your kitchen in weeks. Assume your new kitchen attitude:

1. Walk into the kitchen as you would a job interview. No one needs to know that you're nervous and insecure. All you need to project in the kitchen is confidence.
2. Expect nothing to go as planned.
3. Don't rush yourself (you'll make dumb mistakes and possibly offend anyone who walks into the kitchen). You're not on *Chopped*, and times when I feel like I'm pushed to the wire always go especially terribly.
4. When things don't go as planned, figure out what you can do with what you've got (i.e., turn a failed omelet flip into an egg scramble—no biggie). Rarely does something emerge that's absolutely inedible. I've become damn good at salvaging and transforming first attempts.

Other things to keep in mind:

◆▸ Single attempts are extremely wasteful and inefficient. You bought all the ingredients to make a loaf of bread, and then never use them again; that's the most expensive loaf of bread you've ever bought. On

189

the other hand, making your own bread weekly cuts the cost factor way down since you have all ingredients on hand and now just need to supplement supplies as needed.

- Your success level (and thus confidence) increases when you prepare things in advance, like measuring out your ingredients, cutting your veggies, or washing the pan you'll need in the middle of your recipe. I'm not great at timing, so high levels of preparation help keep me on track.

- You're not alone. There are moms, dads, grandmas, friends, and a whole bunch of strangers to consult (via the interwebs). You're likely not the only person to encounter whatever dilemma it is in which you find yourself, so reach out and use it as a sharing opportunity. Moms love getting phone calls like this—it's an opportunity to help their grown children.

- Give yourself a break. Phase into cooking at home slowly so that a routine shakes out. You're likely to succeed by small, repetitive attempts, not by changing the way you've lived until now in a single day.

phase 1: start your day

Make coffee at home. In eight out of ten cases, you're paying a premium for crappy beans prepared an hour or two in advance, double gross. If you like coffee, not just the idea of coffee (flavored latte, Frappuccino, etc.), set yourself up for home-caffeinated success.

- **Buy decent beans.** This remains the most surefire way to make your own good cup of joe. Paying $10–$15 for a pound of coffee, which will last you for two weeks, is not highway robbery. You're paying $11 a week for a few basic cups of drip coffee in any coffeehouse. If you're truly serious about your cup, look for artisanal roasters who practice direct trade—Stumptown, Intelligentsia, and Counter Culture are great and are available across the country. Remember that a fair trade label guarantees only wages, not bean quality. I don't usually like the mainstream organic/fair trade beans (that's right, I'm a coffee snob, I'll admit it). Give a couple alternative blends a try; you'll find the right ones for your taste buds.

- **Get a grinder.** Don't grind all the beans in advance at the coffeeshop or store; that drains off the freshness and is usually the reason why your coffee at home doesn't taste the same. The aromatic flavor that makes or breaks your coffee starts to go stale the minute you grind it. If your shitty beans don't kill it, pregrinding will.

- Brew with low or no technology via the pour-over method or a French press. You don't need a fancy coffeemaker to enjoy coffeehouse-style cups of coffee every morning.

If you insist on spending money (or brewing espresso), buy a $100-plus grinder before you invest in other coffee technol-

If fancy weekend breakfast projects like pancakes, French toast, or biscuits sound intimidating, try starting out with mixes (pancakes, bread, etc.) to get yourself into the routine.

Once it's normal to be making Sunday brunch at home, expand your experience with made-from-scratch foods.

COOKING AT HOME

ogy. Though we haven't graduated to that level of grind snobbery yet, we still enjoy fine French-press coffee using our small Krups grinder.

Now, for food: what do you eat for breakfast? Think in terms of fuel and grams of protein, the goal for this meal being 15. Keep up the spirit of the Trivial Pursuit game, with extra points for something green for breakfast.

There are all sorts of things you can mix and match in the morning to get you going: eggs, granola (the homemade kind is a fun project), yogurt and cereal, black beans and grits, garden veggies or greens sautéed and served with leftover quinoa from last night's dinner, breakfast tacos, turkey or tofu sausage. The possibilities are endless. Always have a couple options on hand because breakfast monotony is a tedious way to start your day.

phase 2: are those dinner bells?

The momentum builds when you cook at least three dinners at home in a week: your groceries are connected immediately to cooking, which seems like a silly, redundant thing to say, but it's a sad reality that so many times groceries just sit in the fridge as components of meals never made.

solutions:

- **Breakfast for dinner.** Why not? You already have breakfast down, so ritualize omelet or pancake night to shake things up in the evening.
- **Learn some kitchen basics.** It can be from your mom, Netflix (*The French Chef* episodes), YouTube, or whatever, and repeat often. Practice sauté skills, chop-

ping like you mean it, how to poach an egg, whatever eludes you. Adding skills to your kitchen artillery will only give you more options on a night when you're tired and hungry.

→→ **Always make more than you'll eat in one sitting**. This goes for whether you're cooking for yourself or for a whole household. The super-cool thing about making dinner at home is that you've got lunch tomorrow (and maybe extra meals) as an added incentive. Two meals for one night's effort; this is big.

Beyond practicality, cooking at home means you know exactly what you're putting in your body, a luxury not afforded by restaurant cooking. If you're shopping smartly, you know where your vegetables came from, how they were grown, what didn't get injected into your meat. We can't afford to eat regularly at restaurants that pride themselves on that quality (and knowledge about their) fare.

phase 3: experiment with DIY staples

Celebrate your graduation to becoming comfortable using the kitchen by making something that seems fancy. Baking bread is a good example of something you might try to do yourself, but these staples could be any food you buy regularly that probably isn't all that hard to make. Vanilla ice cream has been a fun homemade infusion on our dessert table. See the list at the end of this chapter for more made-from-scratch food inspiration ideas and a bread-from-scratch how-to.

your kitchen toolbox:
where to spend your money

- **A good knife.** A heavy-duty 8-inch chef's knife is the only knife a serious (new) home cook needs to have. The only thing that really matters about your knife is that it feels comfortable and stable in your hand and that it's really sharp (cheap or dull blades are more dangerous since you have to use more force). Expand upon your slicing and dicing repertoire after you know what your real needs are. Are you cutting home-made bread? Are you paring fruit? A note on cost: it's going to run you about $100 if you just go buy it, but sale options are available. I got mine at half off since Wüsthof discontinued the series (the 4587 Grand Prix model). You will need to buy a $30–$40 sharp-ening steel after a year's worth of consistent use with any knife.

- **Rubbermaid high-heat spatula/scraper.** It's white with a red, nylon handle. Buy it online because I've only seen it in stores for $26 (which is less money than you'll pay for dinner for two when you're cooking, by the way). You will use it for everything; I have both the 9.5-inch and 13.5-inch handle lengths and one (or both) is always lurking in my dish-drying rack.

- **Cutting board.** Get at least one that's not a pain in the ass to lug out and clean (translate: not gigantic).

- **A good 10- or 12-inch sauté pan**. I'm anti-nonstick (not down with heating a chemical coating to toxic off-gassing point every day), but do as you please in your house. (Nonstick households have fewer options

194

with cooking tools because you can't use most of your metal utensils on those pots and pans. Teflon flakes in the risotto? No thanks.) I know you have the basic pots and pans, but the great thing about this specific pan is that mostly any meal made in our house can be made in it. As for brand, ours is the 3-quart Calphalon Tri-Ply 18/10 stainless-steel model. It's all metal and can go directly in the oven, which makes it a versatile tool.

- **Two mixing bowls (large- and medium-sized).**
- **A wooden spoon or two.**

Upgrades to make as you can afford them (or find at thrift stores or flea markets):

- **A wire mesh strainer**. I still don't have one, and I kick myself every time I make broth, stock, or jelly.
- **Cooling rack (for bread, cookies, etc.).** After a long time using makeshift cooling racks, this was a super-luxurious addition to my kitchen (for a mere $15).
- **Kitchen scale.** Surprisingly useful, especially in fancier recipes where they call for the weights of ingredients. Recipes using weight also, not surprisingly, tend to have lower failure rates.
- **A set of stainless-steel measuring cups.**

stuck on how to transition your household away from nonstick?

I love these smart, simple tips from the book *Slow Death by Rubber Duck: The Secret Danger of Everyday Things* for prying yourself from reliance upon the off-gassing nonstick cookware:

- Buy a decent skillet/sauté pan. Good choices include cast iron, stainless steel, and enamel-coated cast iron.
- Use enough oil to coat the surface.
- Wait until pan is hot to place food in it.
- Use a metal spatula (not plastic).

195

mis en place

This French term you've probably heard on cooking shows describes the best of intentions, to have all your ingredients gathered and ready in advance.

While this may be crucial for industry chefs, home cooks (like me) might find dinner prep easier (and use considerably less dishes) by preparing as you go. I decide to do this or not do this depending on my mood and time constraints.

These are great if precision matters to you. I still don't own a set, though a ⅓ cup measure would be really helpful.

- **Anything Le Creuset.** Well made, impossible to break, allows food to cook more evenly, and super-versatile in action. Not to mention gorgeous pieces you'll love and treasure forever.
- **A food mill.** If you find yourself jonesing to make applesauce in the fall.

Useless fancy tools, stuff you don't need to buy (even though recipes say you do):

- **Flour sifter.** Use a whisk instead (and the sifter is a complete pain in the ass to clean, by the way).
- **Garlic press.**
- **Mandoline.** Don't get one if you are interested in keeping your fingers.
- **Mini food processor.** Go for the big one, or don't get one at all.
- **Meat tenderizer.**

cookbooks and following recipes

I used to collect cookbooks because I thought that's what every cook should have, a big library of references and resources. Then I realized

Word to the Wise

Newer editions of cookbooks are not always better. I've hoarded a small collection of older editions of *The Joy of Cooking*, since someone thought homemade ice cream and canning and preserving was outdated information around 1970.

that in two years, I hadn't once opened the cookbook cabinet in my single-lady household. I finally realized what the issue was: I'm not good at following recipes.

Cookbooks are super-personal possessions. Any one you actually look in is worth three on the shelf just sitting collecting dust. Prioritize and get acquainted with one cookbook to get yourself started. I accidentally fell in love with *The Joy of Cooking* on a night I couldn't get hold of my mom to ask about cooking temperatures for meats in the middle of dinner preparations. As I flipped through the various sections—meats, vegetables, yeast breads, etc. (all of which are introduced by an overview of methods and useful information)—I discovered Irma's signature recipe formatting (bold print), ingredients in-line with the steps of the preparation method at the spot in which you use them. Who knew a little cut-and-paste action could change my recipe-phobic world entirely: how much you need plus what to do with the ingredient, all in the same place!

I asked my blog readers for the one cookbook they'd choose in a desert island scenario (assuming you had a grocery store on your desert island), and here's what they said:

BASICS:

The Joy of Cooking (of course)
The Way to Cook by Julia Child
Simple Cooking by Alice Waters
The Best Recipe by the editors of *Cooks Illustrated*
Master Recipes by Stephen Schmidt
The Naked Chef Takes Off by Jamie Oliver
The New York Times Cookbook by Craig Claiborne
Better Homes and Gardens New Cookbook, 11th edition

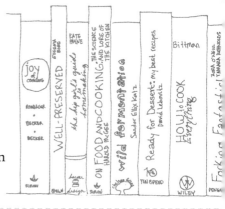

getting the most out of your kitchen ecosystem

- Make stocks from scraps and trimmings. Whip up small batches that you can use within three days, or freeze.
- Buy and roast a whole chicken. This creates many meals, the stock for a soup, and bones for another broth.
- Freeze or preserve fruit you're not going to eat in its prime. Use it in pancakes or muffins.
- Make breadcrumbs from stale bread. Toss the bread in the food processor and freeze the crumbs until needed in a recipe.
- Make your own condiments (mayonnaise, vinaigrette, jams, horseradish, etc.). Not only will you fork over less at the store, but you'll be putting better-quality components in your system.

Ad Hoc at Home by Thomas Keller
How to Cook Everything by Mark Bittman

VEGGIE-STYLE (NOT ONLY FOR VEGETARIANS):

The Modern Vegetarian Kitchen by Peter Berley
Moosewood Restaurant Cooks at Home by the Moosewood Collective
Vegetarian Cooking for Everyone by Deborah Madison
How to Cook Everything Vegetarian by Mark Bittman

Never buy a cookbook before actually perusing it beforehand (either online or at the library) since all recipe authors' styles vary; find the ones you understand and follow most easily. When it comes to buying used copies, any cookbook with Grandma's handwritten notes or recipe cards stashed inside instantly makes my cut, too!

the kitchen ecosystem

"Once you get used to having homemade mayonnaise in the fridge there is no going back to Hellmann's," explains author and savvy chef Eugenia Bone in her *Denver Post* blog, *Preserved* (blogs.denverpost.com/preserved). She coined the term "kitchen ecosystem," and I was lucky enough to spend an enchanted afternoon with her discussing all things kitchen, including efficiency and the small-batch model as well as canning and preserving issues. The more she elaborated on how the kitchen *is* an actual ecosystem, with food in all stages of life and functionality, the more I realized that this is basically permaculture for your kitchen, and any smart, frugal person using common sense will arrive here on her own. Close the loop on wastes, utilize all assets (and forms of food), and insert homemade things as you go (because they're not *that* hard to make).

Things I love about the kitchen ecosystem:

- **It's firmly based in reality, and not theoretical.** Your fridge right now, as is, comprises your ecosystem. You're not working toward anything. You're operating in the everyday realm, making improvements and adding depth as you go.
- **Momentum.** The more you do yourself, from scratch, the more normal that approach becomes. We're so programmed to think that from scratch is harder and thoughtless convenience is better.
- **Having items at "varying stages of utility" in the fridge is an impetus for innovative meal planning and creation.** This is true even for people like me who are actually intimidated by everyday cooking and sustenance.

The possibilities are endless, and they're full of common sense. It's exciting to watch areas of your kitchen unfold with opportunity, such as seeing how to stop stressing over not using groceries how you'd anticipated using them. There are always other ways to extend the life of fresh ingredients or transform marginally good ones into an amazing sauce or soup.

I love this ecosystem idea because it gets to the heart of the

199

matter. As Eugenia wrote, "Thrifty prepping and cooking can get you ahead of the dinner curve in ways that are delicious, conscientious, and uncomplicated."

ap credit: scratch foods

Adding homemade things to your kitchen ecosystem is not only a way to develop richer flavors in meals but also the way to really utilize what you've got. Depending on the tools at hand, the following lists show my favorite things to try doing yourself at least twice (or twelve times), all of which I've managed as a novice. Required tools: just the basic kitchen essentials.

- **Bread.** A weekly task that impresses the pants off everyone who comes in contact with your table.
- **Stovetop popcorn.** Makes you feel like a genius for thwarting the microwave and those handy (and toxic) perfluorocarbon-coated popping bags.
- **Chicken (or vegetable) stock from kitchen scraps.** Inflates your Depression-era-granny ego for making good use of trash (and makes cooking rice the next day flippin' fantastic).
- **Clarified butter.** The single most important thing that has happened to my kitchen thus far. (I suspect mayonnaise will be the next breakthrough.)
- **Pancakes/muffins.** Pancakes remain the best and most impressive brunch-hosting tool ever, and muffins are a quick way to infuse some homemade snackage into your life.
- **Tortillas.** Turning your house into a tortilleria once in a while makes for bad-ass taco nights or (bonus!)

fry up your tortillas into chips. It's the most useful way to rid the fridge of aging tortillas and quell a chips-and-salsa addiction at the same time.

↝ **Make whipped cream.** Pour ½ cup heavy or whipping cream, 1 teaspoon powdered sugar, and a few drops of vanilla extract into a cereal bowl and whisk for a few minutes. You'll thank me when you're dolloping the perfect amount of whipped cream on top of yummy summer fruit (or licking the whisk).

Helpful tool: a good food processor (e.g., a big Cuisinart one or something similar).

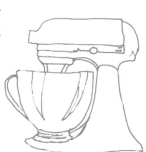

Among the things you can make with it:

↝ Salsa

↝ Smooth soups (like gazpacho or potato leek)

↝ Hummus

↝ Pesto

↝ Pizza dough (fun in the food processor, but works like a charm when hand-kneaded like bread)

↝ Pastry dough

↝ Baby food (or plain vegetable purees you can freeze in ice-cube trays for infusing sauces or baked goods)

Another helpful tool: a fancy stand mixer (e.g., the KitchenAid you received on account of your wedding registry and don't really know what to use it for). It's great for:

↝ Frosting or larger batches of whipped cream

↝ Cakes (and cupcakes)

↝ Cookies

201

- Making homemade butter
- Ice cream (with the ice cream maker attachment; it's the best $50 you'll *ever* spend)

breadwinners can be bread makers too

So I'll admit it: bread making was a stretch, even for me. I didn't really believe in myself, and more important, I liked believing that bread was too tough for me. I was a hard sell until I met an actual dough ball. It was smooshy and stretchy and let me pound and squish and thud out animosities surrounding the Metropolitan Transit Authority or my astonishment at being pelted on the forehead by a seven-year-old with a tangerine. Somewhere between this little yoga workout and the yeast awakening (hellooo, dough puff!) I was sold. I *can* bake bread from scratch.

This might be something your grandma and maybe even your mom did. My store-bought-bread upbringing never really put me in touch with my bread history (my ancestors and their propensities (or aversions) for making bread) nor with my surprising proximity to traditions of bread from scratch.

After looking at too many books and online recipes, I discovered and adapted a recipe that fit two criteria (and my life):

Hip Trick

Keep a kitchen journal. It helps to not only keep track of what you succeed (and fail) at in the kitchen, but also to keep all those things in one place. I keep a small, bound journal and write down ingredient amounts, any improvisations, how much food the recipe made and notes for future attempts. Use a three-ring binder if you like to keep recipes and experiences in an order other than chronological.

1. It didn't intimidate me as a beginning baker.
2. It featured nutritious ingredients found in regular home kitchens (but not too many ingredients).

Simple first, fancy later.

homemade bread for busy people

I know what you're thinking: you have a job, maybe kids, and 237 more pressing things to do than knock off two evenings for bread making. These are more like snippets of evenings, not entire evenings. Hear me out: if I can do this and not hate it, then you can too. If you give it a shot, it will be totally worth it.

Let's talk about the benefits of making bread for a minute:

- There is no one right way to make bread. It's pretty hard to mess it up, and if you do, a toaster and some jam usually fixes the problem.
- You don't need any fancy supplies or expensive equipment. Nope, not even a mixer.
- The slow-rise (arguably best-tasting) method is actually most convenient for busy people.
- Kneading and working with dough is an incredibly satisfying, stress-relieving activity after a long day's work (in nearly all professions, except for maybe bakers).
- Making your own bread is cheaper than purchasing bread of the same nutritional value, and you can avoid all the preservatives and junk in most store-bought bread.
- You get free air freshener by baking at home!

203

even you can make bread

So, I'll admit it, when I first began to make my own bread it was a stretch, even for me. I didn't really believe in myself and, more important, I liked believing that bread was too tough for me. I was a hard sell, until I met an actual dough ball.

It was smooshy and stretchy and let me pound and squish and thud out animosities surrounding the Metropolitan Transit Authority or my astonishment at being pelted on the forehead with an old tangerine by a seven-year-old. Somewhere between this little arm workout and the yeast awakening (hellooo, dough puff!) I was sold. I can bake bread from scratch.

This might be something your grandma and maybe even your mom did. My store-bought wheat bread upbringing never really put me in touch with my bread history—my ancestors and their propensities (or aversions) for making bread—nor my surprising proximity to traditions of making bread from scratch.

There are no less than 500 ways to make the same thing (bread), so I don't blame you for feeling overwhelmed by the prospect. Visit the Hip Girl's Guide to Homemaking blog for my tried-and-true recipes and methods for simple honey wheat sandwich bread or my signature gluten-free millet oat bread for both oven and bread machine preparation.

But first, here's a quick rundown on the ins and outs of bread. Bread may seem like a lot of steps at first, but as you become familiar with the phases, you'll be able to fold it into your routine.

eight fun things you can do with a loaf of your homemade bread

1. Eat all of it immediately.

2. Invite friends to your house for a tea party, where you chat with mouths full of cucumber sandwiches on homemade deliciousness.

3. Send a loaf to your granny, who loves getting packages and quite likely doesn't bother with the "hassle" of fresh loaves any longer.

4. Make caprese bites (or some other zesty little appetizer) and bring them to a dinner party or potluck.

5. Bring freshly baked bread to new friends who showed you how to do something. I brought a hunk of crusty wonderfulness as a gesture of thanks to friends who showed me how to can tomatoes. Tit for tat.

6. Take a loaf to your new neighbors. Get tight with the people who live on top of, beside, or below you.

7. Bread makes a perfect gift for people going through times of transition: births, deaths, surgeries, and everything in between. Everyone's gotta eat; why not provide fresh warm bread?

8. Kick-ass French toast. 'Nuff said.

yeast breads

When you bake bread, most recipes call for yeast. (Quick breads are those recipes that utilize baking soda and/or powder instead of yeast to puff up the dough.)

Active dry yeast is the most common kind you'll probably use and it comes in packet form for easy portioning. This kind of yeast needs water and a little bit of sugar to activate. The cool thing about mastering yeast is that once you get it, you'll gain access to other cool homemade projects like bagels, pizza dough, and doughnuts!

wet vs. dry ingredients

Usually you'll combine wet and dry ingredients in separate bowls and then gradually add the dry to the wet to form your dough. This ensures an even distribution of ingredients.

knead

Kneading your dough allows the flour to develop its gluten "muscle" strength. As you work your dough, it will become stretchy and more elastic—a perfect shell to house millions of yeast-produced carbon dioxide pockets. Yum. Gluten-free breads will develop their elasticity in the mixer or in your mixing bowl.

Kneading is easy. There's a little method involved, but you may personalize your kneading style as you get more practice. Tips for easy kneading:

1. Dust a little flour on a clean countertop. Flatten your dough with the heel of your hands (lower palms) and then fold the dough over itself (like a taco).
2. Work it flat again and then rotate the flat pancake a quarter turn and repeat the taco roll and flatten again.

206

3. Every now and then pick the dough up and slam it down on the counter with a big whack!

rise

Most yeast breads need two opportunities to rise, one to develop gluten strength fully, and the other to prepare the bread for baking. Gluten-free bread bakers need only provide one rise since alternative grains' protein molecules behave differently from those of wheat.

By the time this stage appears you have a pile of dirty dishes (a mixing bowl and measuring cups and spoons) staring at you from the sink. I only have one large mixing bowl, so at this point I have to wash it. Don't forget to grease the bowl before you set dough in for the rise. (I learned this lesson the hard way!)

For best rise results, cover dough with a slightly damp tea towel or greased plastic wrap and stick the loaf pans in a cool oven, keeping the oven off. The pilot light (if you have a gas oven) creates the perfect temp for the final rise. (My house is chilly in the winter and the open countertop doesn't work well for the final rise.) If your house is not gas powered, turn the oven on, let it reach 200°F and then turn it off. Stick the dough ball in after the oven has been off for at least 10 minutes.

For those of you with instructions for two rises, the second one happens in the loaf pan or in whatever baking medium you choose. You'll punch down the dough, place it in the pans and get it ready to bake by leaving it alone for a while. Lots

Hip Trick

You can always double a bread recipe by following it through the first rise and then sticking extra dough balls in the fridge for quick homemade bread during the next month. Don't forget to date your dough bags.

To defrost, just place the balls in the fridge until thawed and then follow your recipe's instructions for the second rise.

of breaks mean you can accomplish other things during your bread-making session.

bake

Ovens vary in temperature and heating patterns, so rotating your loaf pans midway through the baking time will ensure the loaves are cooked uniformly.

To test for doneness, I stick my thermometer in the corner of the near-finished loaf just to be sure my oven hasn't gone wild. Take the loaves out when the thermometer reads 200–205 degrees internally. Drop your loaves out of the pans immediately and place them to cool on the rack. Note the hollow sound when you tap the bottom of the loaves as this is another sign of doneness.

the perfect crust

My first few loaves left a lot to be desired in the crust category. Here are a couple ways to darken your crust:

1. Place a small (oven-safe) pot or pan on the bottom rack of the oven before turning it on and then add one cup of water three minutes before you put your loaf in to bake. Be extremely careful; the initial steam produced by pouring in the water can burn you!

Hip Trick

My favorite way to store homemade bread is wrapped in waxed paper as tightly as you can manage and leave it on the counter. We tie our loaves up with kitchen twine for easy access and resealing capabilities.

The fridge dries out bread fast, so avoid keeping it in there.

2. Brush the loaf top with melted butter or a well-whisked egg.

first-timer tips

It's important to make baking special, not stressful. Here are a few tips and words of advice for you to keep in mind:

1. Though any day will do in the future; give yourself some room on the first attempt. Select a day where you're not in a time crunch, perhaps a lazy weekend afternoon.
2. Phone a friend. Said friend does not actually have to be involved in the baking process, but you need a warm body in the room. This person will be invaluable in helping you to not take yourself so seriously and keeping flour out of the computer keyboard if you're following an online recipe.
3. Read the recipe all the way through before you start. Map out the waiting periods and determine if you have enough time from start to finish. You don't want to be up until 2:30 a.m. waiting to pull your loaves out of the oven, trust me.
4. Recipes are meant to be broken. I'm directions-phobic; give me a set of instructions and I'll start devising a way of altering or avoiding them. Give yourself some room to interpret one person's method into one that works well for you.
5. Clean and sanitize your countertop before getting started so you don't have to worry about it while you're

elbow deep in flour and transitioning from mixing to kneading.

6. Don't try to knead your dough on a cutting board, no matter the size or material. Unless your board has industrial-strength suction cups, you'll end up frustrated.

7. Make tea (or margaritas) to make it official; a drink of some sort helps you remember that you are having fun. A pretty apron helps too.

8. Don't cut the finished product until it has cooled completely (approximately 40 minutes) since it is still developing flavor in the cooling process.

9. Relax! Don't give yourself a hard time about perfection. So, your first shot didn't place you in the running for the best up-and-coming artisan baker awards. Bread making begs you to simply live and learn. It's really hard to make bread that's entirely inedible. After all, dense bread still tastes like homemade bread, and makes a pretty kick-ass French toast.

resources

books

- → *The Omnivore's Dilemma* by Michael Pollan.
  Will change the way you view food and wandering around the grocery store.
- → *Something from the Oven* by Laura Shapiro.
  Covers the rise of the food industry, why popular food became so gross in the 1950s, roles of women and domesticity, feminism, and general inspiration.

- *On Food and Cooking* by Harold McGee.
  Demystifies chemical and physical properties of food and helps you understand why certain things behave the way they do in the kitchen.

- *The Sharing Solution: How to Save Money, Simplify Your Life and Build Community* by Janelle Orsi and Emily Doskow.
  Will help you start a buying club or think up other ways to collectively save money on food with your neighbors, friends, or community.

web

- localharvest.org
  Find local farmers' markets, nearby CSAs, and real food resources

chapter 9

preserving food at home

stock your pantry with a new kind of convenience

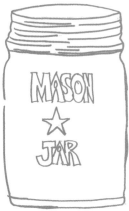

Don't worry, this chapter spares you the pastoral portrait that usually accompanies the subject matter, mainly because I don't have any nostalgic stories to relay. No cute grannies in the kitchen hovering over pots. No childhood spent lounging under apple trees (though I did have a grapefruit tree fort). When I began this book a year ago, I had never seen anyone can anything, and I had minimal experience eating such treats.

I'm not complaining. Actually, Bertha Burnham (my not-so-domestic gram) made blackberry jam once. She laughed as she recalled how the jam didn't set (pectin problems), but they ate the failed syrupy jam all winter long over ice cream. Not too shabby.

Over the past year, I've taken a number of classes (including an online home food preservation course through the University of Georgia) and apprenticed with expert canners to get a grasp on the ins and outs of this cool science-project-turned-impressive-kitchen-trick. I now lead classes in my home and at food events for beginning canners.

Of the many ways to preserve food, water bath and pressure canning get the most attention and heat. You can preserve just about any kind of food using these two methods (some things, like all low-acid foods, may only be pressure-canned). In this chapter we'll start with the preservation that you already do, involving the fridge and freezer, and then help you ease into the idea that canning is not beyond your capacities.

I'm not going to even try to be a comprehensive how-to resource on this subject. There's so much to cover and so many other books and websites already do it well (see resources at the end of this chapter). I'll defer to that excellent body of knowledge out there to steer you along the path of safe home preserving. I have included the things that most of those sources omit, the things that make first-time canners spend way too much time Googling and pulling their hair out.

I was in contact with Eugenia Bone as I wrote this chapter; she's a master canner and one of the only authors of canning lit I've encountered who has her feet firmly planted in reality. She took the fear and mystery out of canning both in her book and in person. If you enjoy the magic factor that is a standard Ball book recipe, then by all means can away in magicland, but as you encounter real-life situations and ingredient scenarios that arise, a little practicality (and science explained) is a welcome treat.

preserving your sanity

Most of us don't live on the prairie; we're not putting up an entire harvest's worth of fruit and veggies. You are not likely to starve over the winter if you don't can.

You're buying as much seasonal food as you can afford (or grow on your back deck) and eating as much of it as possible fresh, and if there's anything left, hopefully stashing some away for later. If you want to do full-day canning sessions with bushels and crates of produce, be my guest, but incorporating modes of smaller-scale preservation into your existing routine is a more sustainable route for your sanity's sake. By putting aside (in the freezer or in a jar) some of what you buy or what you make for one dinner, you're spreading your resources out efficiently. When tomato and apple seasons roll around, you'll get the chance to decide how you feel about the all-day canning affair.

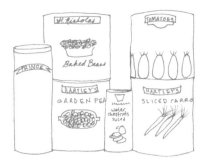

DIY **convenience**

Homemade convenience products may sound like an oxymoron. If you're wondering why you might consider filling your own jars rather than letting people you don't know do it for you, here are a few reasons:

- ▸ Knowing where your food comes from and what's really in it is the best kind of health insurance you can buy (or make).
- ▸ Eating local produce all year round (thanks to jars and hot water) supports your regional food system.
- ▸ Homemade convenience is flat-out impressive and richens your kitchen's ecosystem—pestos to develop flavor in plain old pasta, preserved lemons added to a salmon marinade, canned plums to add to baked goods, and pancakes all winter long.
- ▸ You'll have goods on hand to give as birthday and holiday gifts or to trade at food swaps.
- ▸ It extends the season for food you can't get enough of.

Making your own convenience and everyday products puts you back in charge of what you put in your body. Plus it positions you to better enjoy the real joy of cooking: not having to go to the store for every ingredient in a recipe.

Word to the Wise

A general rule of thumb for refrigerator storage of cooked leftovers is absolutely no more than three days. If you can't remember how long it's been in there, throw it out.

where to start

Start with the foods you actually eat. Whatever excites you is the most logical entrance to canning and preserving. That will dictate the method and equipment you focus on. Your next step should be to identify things that will improve things you already make.

What do you eat at night? For breakfast? First things first, go to your pantry and fridge right now and see what types of store-bought canned goods you already have.

The time to can something is not when it's wilting and on the edge of the produce/compost zone. You should can produce that's as fresh and close to harvest as possible. Like with most systems, your outputs are only as good as your inputs. Boiling something, while it kills the things that cause spoilage, will not do any flavor favors for less-than-ideal produce. Instead, use your wilting veggies to make stocks.

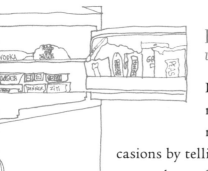

preservation you already do
uncharted territory: your refrigerator

I've had a turbulent relationship with my refrigerator over the years. I horrified my mother on numerous occasions by telling her about leftovers I'd consumed many days after even liberal recommendations passed. As a result of marginal leftover consumption, I've had my share's worth of food poisoning, which is no fun.

It's probably not surprising, my obsession with wanting to know exactly how long things keep in the fridge. My mom, tired of hearing me groan about tummy troubles, says forty-eight hours; the USDA says seventy-two. I can handle this range.

A quick food safety primer:

- Keep hot food hot and cold food cold. You get a two-hour window (one hour if food is sitting out when it's above 90°F) to transport or safely eat foods before spoilers can bloom.
- There are two kinds of spoilers in food. *Spoilage bacteria* are behind the natural method of food decomposition that causes food to go bad. Food looks and smells funny (or gross), which makes the food unappealing but not necessarily harmful. *Pathogenic bacteria* are the ones that make you sick (foodborne illness, commonly referred to as food poisoning). You can't see, smell, or taste these bacteria. (And, by the way, mold is not bacteria. Molds and yeasts are both fungi naturally occurring in foods and are destroyed at temperatures between 140°F and 190°F. Mold requires air, food, and moisture to thrive.)

If you have specific questions about what's safe in the fridge, consult the USDA Food Safety Education website, fsis.usda.gov /Food_Safety_Education/index.asp; the fact sheets are a great resource.

Hip Trick

I've had an embarrassing amount of experience with food poisoning (that is, before the universal law of leftovers truly set in for me). If you're tender-bellied (or have plans to travel somewhere iffy) buy a small bottle of Oreganol and keep it with you. It shouldn't cost more than $20 and it'll last forever. Three drops of the super-potent oil in a small glass of water or juice will knock out any unusual suspects in your stomach.

the frozen tundra: your freezer

I know you have a freezer. It probably has frozen peas, a bottle of vodka, and maybe some batteries in it. Or it's quite possibly stocked so full that you have no clue what's really inside those foil-wrapped packages and mysterious freezer bags. Either scenario is not particularly helpful to you.

The freezer can be a really useful tool in stashing excess, both already cooked leftovers and ready-to-cook fruits, vegetables, and meats. When it comes to successful freezing, excess moisture is enemy number one (and usually the reason your freezing endeavors fail). Excessively watery things like leafy greens, potatoes, and milk products balloon up with ice crystals in the freezing process. When thawed, their cell walls, stretched and destroyed, reflect this ballooning, leaving these kinds of things limp, lifeless, or undesirably chunky.

put a lid on it

Freezing halts spoilage by removing liquid water from the cells of the food and replacing it with ice crystals. When considering what to freeze, the question is quality, not safety. Successful freezing minimizes opportunities for large ice crystals, which deteriorate the quality of your food, to form.

Keeping foods in as airless a package as possible is your best bet for avoiding freezer burn. This is why you don't want to use the standard (not freezer-quality) plastic bags or standard pop-on lid Tupperware containers (without added protections) for longer-term freezing.

Here are a few tips on how to freeze stuff so you actually want to eat it later.

avoid freezing these items or leftovers that contain them

- Potatoes (mashed or whole).
- Leafy greens (though my mom is on a successful chives freezing spree; she uses the thawed chives in things where a limp chive won't make a difference, like mashed potatoes or in soups).
- Cucumbers, radishes, and cabbage.
- Milk products.
- Whole eggs. You can separate and freeze whites, because they freeze well alone. Or beat together the yolk and white, add a little salt or sugar, and freeze it.
- Cooked pasta and rice. Only cook enough for one meal at a time; frozen-and-thawed versions end up mushy and lifeless.

219

what is blanching and why do we do it?

Blanching involves dipping vegetables in boiling water for a minute or two and then transferring them to an ice water bath before sealing for freezing. The boiling water inactivates enzymes that affect color and the breakdown of vitamins, and the ice water dip stops further cooking and damage to cell walls. Thus blanching helps keep foods true to their original color, and retain nutritional value when frozen.

→ Use rigid, airtight containers made of glass or plastic for the freezer. (Most standard plastic Tupperware and take-out containers are not airtight, but a layer of plastic wrap placed on top of the food before adding the lid can help minimize the food's contact with freezer air.)

→ Any straight-sided canning jar can be used for freezing. Wide-mouth pint or half-pint jars are the best since contents can expand evenly upward during crystallization. (The regular-mouth jars that have a smaller rim than body can break when contents expand inside.) Leave at least an inch of head space when filling the jar with food, and leave the lid loose for the first few hours in the freezer. I broke a few too many glass jars before I finally learned this lesson.

→ Some foods (many fruits and small-kernel vegetables) benefit from a quick, container-less freeze on a cookie sheet and then should be placed in airtight, moisture-resistant containers. This allows the ice crystals to form evenly around individual berries or kernels and minimizes damage to the cell walls when thawed.

→ Have a stash of quart-sized plastic freezer bags on hand. Gallon-sized bags are handy for loaves of bread and larger quantities of

220

fruits and vegetables. Reusing freezer bags for other areas of the house is fine, but try to stick with only new bags when freezing food directly in them. (Normal wear and tear creates small holes in bags and increases the chances of freezer burn.)

- Double up protection when freezing something in laminated paper, like your butcher-paper-wrapped hamburger meat, by wrapping it in foil or placing it in a freezer bag.
- Lightweight aluminum foil is generally inadequate for home freezing; look for brands labeled for freezing.
- Divide up large portions of food (soups, casseroles, meat roasts) into smaller containers for freezing. Cool food in the refrigerator before placing it in the freezer; this will keep ice crystals small when you eventually place it in the freezer.
- Don't forget to label your frozen goodies with contents and date. It doesn't take long to completely forget what's in those frosty little containers tucked in every nook and cranny.

General rules for freezing common foods:

- **Fruit.** Space apart on a cookie sheet and freeze for ten minutes, then throw into freezer bags once frozen. Keep no longer than six to eight months for best quality.
- **Vegetables.** Blanch the vegetables (see sidebar), then dry them completely. Freeze in small portions for use.

Hip Trick

Grandma Mannie told me her favorite way to eat summer corn all winter long is to buy a bunch of it at the farm stand or market, boil it as you would if you were eating it right away, cut it off the cob, and place the kernels into freezer bags in dinner-sized servings. All you have to do is pull out a bag and heat it up to enjoy summer's tastiest treat even when it's snowing outside.

When you thaw something in the fridge, be sure to set it in an empty bowl as a precautionary measure for when its ice melts. A puddle or tidal wave in the fridge is not a useful addition to your kitchen ecosystem.

Keep no longer than six months to one year for best quality.

- **Meats.** Large packages of fresh meat may be broken down into dinner-sized portions, or double-wrap the existing package of already-portioned meat products. Keeps no longer than four to nine months. Thawed meat will lose liquid fast when cooked, so longer cooking times at lower temperatures are better for retaining moisture.

- **Bread.** Wrap a completely cooled loaf in foil and place in a freezer bag. We slice our bread before freezing so it's easy to grab a few slices at a time for breakfast toast or sandwiches. (With only two of us in the house it's hard for us to eat an entire loaf in the two to four days before it gets stale on the countertop.)

The National Center for Home Food Preservation website (see "Resources" in this chapter) has detailed guidelines on how to freeze specific ingredients and food items properly.

bringing food back up to speed

- Reheat leftovers at 165°F to safely kill any bacteria that may have formed in the fridge (this won't happen in the freezer). As you might remember from Chapter 1, we are a non-microwave household. Our toaster oven and range top get a lot of action.

- If you didn't have the foresight to thaw your dinner in advance (by placing it in the refrigerator until it thaws,

eight smart things to freeze

1. Meat bones from individual dinners to make stock when you have enough of them stashed, and then any leftover stock you can't use within three days.

2. Homemade bread crumbs from stale bread.

3. Coffee, tea (both cooled in the refrigerator first), and syrup from fruit preserves in ice cube trays; they make fun additions to beverages or tasty mini ice pops.

4. Excess pesto, also placed in ice cube trays to freeze (then stored in freezer bags). Pop one out for some homegrown basil pizzazz at the height of winter drear.

5. Dinner-sized portions of precooked meals, a tool that will save money—and your sanity—during busy workweeks. I like to freeze future dinners right away since you might not get to the meals before it goes bad in the fridge (and I hate fridge guilt).

6. An extra jar of preserves or jam you made but didn't process in the water bath (see recipe later on in the chapter).

7. A ball of bread dough in between its first and second rises. You got hip to doubling the batch during busy weeks in the last chapter. Thaw it in the fridge, set it out to let it rise again, and then bake. Plan-ahead bread!

8. Corn flour (masa), whole-wheat flour, or any other flour with high oil content (ones that include the bran and the germ). Freezing keeps them from going rancid, and the added heft of dry grains/flours helps the freezer retain cold better than empty air. You'll save money on your electric bill and free up room in your pantry.

which is the best method), then place the food in an airtight bag (translate: any new plastic bag that seals with a zipper or slider) and run it under cold water until it's ready to be reheated on the stove. Or just take the food out of its freezer container, put it in an oven-safe pot, stick it in the oven, and heat at a low temperature (250°F) until the food reaches 165°F. Eat promptly.

i will never can

I dedicate this section to my mom, nearly all my good friends, and anyone who's ever uttered those four words. Convincing yourself that canning is not too involved is perhaps the biggest challenge you'll face.

I've picked a few sweet and savory ways to eat your way through the seasons (and beyond) that you don't have to process in a water bath canner. But first, let's cover some basics of hygiene and bust your sterilization myth fears.

Even though you don't have to process the jars—which tends to spook most potential canners—you might consider sterilizing the jars for these three recipes. You'll want hot jars for packing hot food in them in the case of the rhubarb and pickle recipes, and you'll prevent any potential spoilers from decreasing the fridge life of your goods.

preserved lemons: stashing winter's harvest

I took a chance on these. When I first entered my Meyer lemon craze—when they appeared during winter months at my co-op—I hadn't a clue how we would use preserved lemons. But they smelled so good that I compulsively bought as many as would fit into my bag on every grocery-acquisition occasion. Sometimes the most fun part of preserving food is the forced expansion of taste and utility.

Preserved lemons are a staple in Moroccan cuisine, which we rarely make or eat, but it turns out the intense lemon burst improves everything that touches our table. We use them in salad dressing or for an infusion of flavor in a meat, fish, or vegetable dish.

This is a great first-timer activity because preserving Meyer lemons is so easy, and the lemons are so acidic that it's impossible to grow any unwanted toxins in the jar.

preserved meyer lemons

Meyer lemons are über-fragrant natives of China; they're a cross between a mandarin orange and a lemon. The skin is softer than traditional lemons, and pleasantly edible. Meyer lemons are grown in the United States' more tropical regions (California, Texas, and Florida) between November and March. If you don't see any in your local grocery during these times, you can always use any organic lemon; just grab a few extra for juicing, since they're not nearly as juicy as Meyers.

This recipe comes from Eugenia Bone's book *Well-Preserved: Recipes*

hip trick

Vacuum-seal meat you want to freeze by submerging the filled freezer bag in a bowl of room temperature water (maybe the water you used to wash your lettuce or other produce) and being careful to not let water seep into the top of the bag.

I recommend only using new freezer bags for this, or slight holes that result from wear will let water (and freezer air) into your bag.

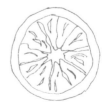

and *Techniques for Putting Up Small Batches of Seasonal Foods* and yields 2 pints.

Here's what you need:

10 Meyer lemons
½ cup kosher salt
2 wide-mouth pint mason jars or volume-equivalent smaller jars

1. Sterilize your jars by bringing them to a boil in a pot that will allow them to be submerged. Boil for 10 minutes.
2. Simmer (not boil) two new mason jar lids. This warms up the gummy seal stuff.
3. Slice stem ends from 6 lemons and quarter lengthwise from pole to pole.
4. Juice remaining 4 lemons.
5. Distribute lemons between the two still-hot jars, interspersing 3 Tablespoons kosher salt into each jar. Don't pulverize the lemons getting them in the jar, but really do pack them down. You don't want air pockets between the lemons.
6. Top off jars with lemon juice, leaving about ½ inch head space. Your lemons should be mostly submerged.
7. Add 1 Tablespoon more of salt to both jars.
8. Wipe rims of jars clean with a clean, damp cloth. Lid the jars and place them on your countertop to develop brine for two weeks. Invert jars every other day to keep salt evenly distributed.

After two weeks on the counter, put jars in the fridge to halt the fermentation process. Use within six months for best flavor, but they will keep for up to a year in the fridge.

sweet preserves:
spreading spring on toast

Making a small batch of preserves or jam to eat over the next few weeks is not unlike the act of buying a (pricey) jar of jam at the store. How often do you buy a jar of jam to keep indefinitely on the pantry shelf? You buy it to eat it; duh. Once you open it, your jar of jam has a number of weeks (sometimes more than a month) in the fridge until the fuzzies appear.

You can make any jam, jelly, preserves, or other sweet spread without canning it in a water bath. The first step, cooking the fruit and getting it to gel, is completely independent of the water bath processing step (the way to hermetically seal the jar and keep it stashed on the pantry shelf, which I describe later in this chapter).

This super-small-batch method is perfect for when finances restrict you from buying more than a pound of produce at the market, when your home harvest is small (kudos to all the rhubarb home growers out there), or for previewing flavors in a spread you might want to make in larger quantities later. Your jam or sweet spread will be the better for it, since you're only boiling your tender fruit once. And a homemade luxury item is wildly impressive to whip out the next time your pals come over for drinks.

how to sterilize a jar

Pop it in the dishwasher with the heated dry cycle selected

or

Boil it for 10 minutes in a stockpot that allows for water to reach the tops of the jars (and not boil over the edge and onto your range top).

227

rhubarb hibiscus vanilla preserves

This is a two-day recipe, which is actually easier for busy people to incorporate into their schedules. The first slot involves preparing the produce and can be done in the evening or in the morning, and the second part just involves cooking the fruit for all of 15 minutes. That's it. You'll get about 1 pint.

Cut into ½-inch cross-sections (of stalk) **1 pound rhubarb** (which ends up being about 2½ cups) and place in a heavy-bottomed pot.

Add:

1½ cups granulated sugar (raw is fine)

⅓ cup dried whole hibiscus flowers, chopped into small pieces

Scrape seeds into the pot from:

½ vanilla bean, sliced lengthwise (if you can't find a vanilla bean use ¼ teaspoon of a pure vanilla extract or just skip it) and toss bean pod into the pot. Cover with lid and let fruit macerate (fancy word for let the sugar break down the fruit a bit) overnight or for at least 6 hours. If you are using vanilla extract skip it here; you'll add it after you cook the preserves.

When you return to the pot, most of the sugar will be dissolved. Add **1 Tablespoon strained lemon juice** (about half a small lemon) and place mixture over medium heat to dissolve any remaining sugar. Stir with a good rubber spatula (or wooden spoon) to keep sugar from scorching the bottom of the pan. Bring to a boil.

Once the mixture is boiling, it will take about 10 minutes for it to thicken up. Once that happens, remove the pan from the heat and let it sit for 5 minutes before ladling it into a hot pint jar (or two half-pint jars). If you're using vanilla extract, add it just before you put the mixture in the jars.

Stick the jar in the fridge after it has cooled for an hour on the counter.

(If you want to water bath can this, you may double the recipe [or not] and process jars for 15 minutes in water bath canner. This is the one instance where it's okay to double a sweet spread recipe, since I wrote it as a super-small batch. Don't increase it beyond double though because otherwise it may not gel properly.)

fridge pickles: crunch your way through summer

Unless you have a whole plot's worth of cukes (or some other vegetable that appeared en masse in your CSA share), small batches of fresh pickles are ideal for fridge storage. In most cases you have room for the small yields—three pints or a couple quart jars, at most—and you probably already have a few jars of store-bought pickles taking up real estate. Evict these lowly tenants and replace them with home-pickled equivalents.

Making fresh pickles (by that I mean not fermented) is pretty easy. You've already mastered the skill set if you can successfully bring anything to a boil.

dill pickled cukes

Modified from Linda Ziedrich's book *The Joy of Pickling: 250 Flavor-Packed Recipes for Vegetables and More From Garden or Market*
Yields 1 quart
Instructions:

Place in a clean, quart-sized mason jar:

8 whole black peppercorns

2 cloves garlic, chopped

2 dried hot peppers (usually found in spice or ethnic food section of your grocery)

2 teaspoons dried dill seeds (or 3 to 4 fesh dill fronds)

Pack **about 1¹⁄₃ pounds of Kirby (4-inch pickling cucumbers), halved, quartered, or kept whole** into the jar; this is really just as many as you can fit in there, so weight doesn't ultimately matter. It's handy to pack most of your cukes in vertically and then position a few pieces horizontally over the top to "seatbelt" (term and idea courtesy of WellPreserved.ca bloggers Dana and Joel, not to be confused with the book Eugenia Bone wrote!) the cukes in and keep them from bobbing up out of the vinegar brine.

Combine in a stainless steel saucepan and bring to boil to dissolve salt:

1 cup water

1 cup white wine vinegar (distilled white vinegar is okay, too)

1 Tablespoon pickling or Kosher salt

Remove liquid mixture from heat and pour it into your cucumber-packed jar leaving ½-inch of space from the top rim of the jar. If your brine doesn't cover the top of your cukes, just top it off with water (this is safe to do here because you're just fridge pickling and thus don't need to worry about the acidity level in the jar).

Wipe any vinegar spills from the rim of the jar, throw a lid on it and hide it from yourself in the back of your fridge for a couple weeks (or until you can't stand to wait any longer) and try to eat them within six months. We're lucky if they last a week after we crack them open in our house.

putting up

I didn't grow up canning food (or "putting up," as some canners call it), and up until a year ago I had never even seen anyone do it. It's initially mysterious and potentially dangerous if done haphazardly. I decided that my first exposure should be through participant observation. I was a newcomer to NYC, so I resorted to the Internet.

Social media outlets like Twitter and Facebook are probably the last places you'd think to look for the how-to on canning and preserving food. After nearly a week with zero response to my emails, tweets, Facebook pleas, and even Craigslist ads, I began to assume that everyone who cans at home must live on the West Coast, or somewhere that's not New York. I was discouraged by the overwhelming nonresponse until I got a single tweet from a guy who had pickle pride (and not so much the urge to invite a stranger over for 5 hours on the weekend).

I proceeded to do what any Internet stalker might do: I checked out his Twitter profile and Googled him. Then I emailed him. Telling him about myself, my project, and my previous experience with anthropological fieldwork was my best attempt at climbing from the rank of "demanding stranger" to "invited guest" at his next canning session. Also, this follow-through takes social media from the limited, faceless arena into the realm of true human community.

After a couple more emails and his discussion with the "canner in chief," his wife (which I'd have given anything to hear:

231

"Honey, so remember how I have a Twitter account . . . ?"), I was sitting at a kitchen table with my new friends, just five or six days after our first noncommittal, faceless interaction.

If I could find the one pickler in NYC who was (sort of) willing to welcome me into his home, surely you can find someone near you who's putting food up. Take a class if it makes you feel better, but it's not required. You just need to see someone actually doing it to remove some of the fear and stigma loaded into home food preservation.

botulism blows

Your first question is about botulism, I know. Botulism, the disease caused by the bacteria *Clostridium botulinum*, is the main reason why more people aren't running to the hardware store to buy $12 worth of supplies to put up big or small batches of seasonal foods to enjoy all year long.

The canning literature doesn't do much to reassure people; the pervading theme of introduction-to-canning books is usually "Follow these rules exactly or you'll die." Truth is, you're probably more likely to have a run-in with botulism if you keep garlic suspended in olive oil in a jar on the counter, or let baked potatoes come to room temperature wrapped in aluminum foil.

Roughly twenty-two cases of botulism are reported in the United States per year from foodborne sources, according to the Centers for Disease Control and Prevention, many of which result from unsafe kitchen practices such as those mentioned in the paragraph above. I'm not taking this risk lightly by any means, but once you understand the precise scientific conditions required to activate *Clostridium botulinum* spores, the fear becomes more manageable. The bacteria spores need all of the following five conditions to activate and release the toxin into your food:

1. Anaerobic (airless) environment
2. Low acid level (a pH above 4.6)
3. Higher temperatures (usually higher within the "danger zone," which is 40–140°F)
4. Moisture
5. Food

Doing the opposite of any of these will inhibit activation of the toxin spores. In many cases you've hermetically sealed a high-acid mixture (most fruits have a lower pH than 4.6, and all pickles are acidified to below 4.6), and botulism can't activate there, period. If you should have any questions about your pressure-canned low-acid foods, just boil the food for ten minutes before eating it to ensure safety. Or you can always place anything that's questionable (or that doesn't seal) directly into the fridge within a couple hours of processing.

water bath canning

This method hermetically seals jars through the ingenious use of boiling water. You already know that you don't have to can it if you don't intend to store it on the shelf, but if your fridge is full or if you want to make a bunch of shippable holiday presents, you'll need to process the jars in a water bath.

The natural, normal spoilage of fresh produce is caused by microorganisms, which are present in large numbers in foods as well as in the air. Processing the jar destroys these spoilage microorganisms and, as previously mentioned, the only foods

233

you can in a water bath are high-acid things, so the bacteria that causes botulism can't germinate. The jar is sealed off from the surrounding air by means of the rubber flange on the lid (of most kinds of jars) and secured in place by a band.

Hip Trick

A pressure canner is a great thing to purchase with one or two friends. A new Presto brand pressure canner runs about $80 (and is well worth the investment when split two or three ways). You'll save money and have it when you really need it (and get it out of the way when you don't).

Creating higher-than-normal pressure in the jar forces hot air, steam, and possibly small amounts of liquid out of the jar from under the lid. This is a one-way process, out; the lid and rim do not allow air and cooking water to enter the jar from the outside. As the jar cools down after processing, a vacuum is created inside.

You can store this hermetically sealed jar on the shelf for up to a year, if you can manage not eating it for that long!

pressure canning

This is the method for killing microorganisms in low-acid environments via steam. I only do it with friends because I don't have my own pressure canner, yet. A pressure canner is a special piece of equipment you'll need to buy if you envision canning meats, broths, beans, vegetables (that aren't acidified with vinegar), lemon curd, or other low-acid foods that need to be brought to temperatures higher than water bath canning allows for. *Never* attempt to water bath can these kinds of foods; utilize other methods of preserving, like freezing, if you don't have a pressure canner.

There are two kinds of pressure canners, a dial gauge or a

weighted gauge; both types have clamps that lock the canner, a way to measure steam pressure inside, and safely release the steam should the pressure become too heavy. The temperature inside a locked and properly operated pressure canner reaches above 240°F and successfully kills both spoilers that made their way into your packed jars and the dormant form (spores) of the bacteria that cause botulism.

essential tools

- **Thermometer.** I've had a hell of a time with cheap thermometers. My mom gave me a high-end digital one and I don't think twice about it now; you can find a decent one for under $30 (try Taylor Precision products). That said, I survived and managed just fine without a fancy one for a whole year of cooking, canning, and bread making. Marisa, my friend who writes the *Food in Jars* blog, swears by her Taylor Pro Series combination thermometer/timer with a 4-foot-long probe; you can let the probe sit in the bubbling mixture on the stove and not burn your fingers.

- **Kitchen scale.** I held out the longest on this one. The immediate gains from precision were lost on me, but I soon learned how helpful it is to not have to scout out equivalents online every time I prepare (or reduce) a recipe. Once purchased, it's one of those appliances that you're not quite sure how you got along without. Plus you can use your scale in baking recipes posted by weight. I'm not a real exactness monger, but an enhanced level of precision will serve as an additional buffer against failure.

235

- **Stock pot.** Don't buy a galvanized metal canner kit. You can't cook anything else in that galvanized ordeal, and single-purpose kitchen equipment is really dumb. If you don't already have one, scout out a good bargain on Craigslist (where I bought my 10-gallon enameled steel lobster pot). You can use any size pot, though, that fits your desired jar size, which is handy for smaller batches. But if you have the choice, taller is better since you want jars to be submerged in at least a couple of inches of water, and you don't want the water to boil over the top.

- **Rack.** This will depend on the size of your stock pot. If you bought a lobster pot (or any other big-ass stock pot), then grab the traditional canning rack with handles (a useful feature for finding sterilized, clear jars in a vat of boiling water). If you have a smaller pot, then buy a cake or pie cooling rack just smaller in diameter than your pot. Or instead of a rack, try a collapsible steamer basket or canner lids hooked together with kitchen twine.

- **Jars.** Start out by using Ball or Kerr jars with two-piece lids; you can graduate to experimenting with Weck or single-piece lids after you get the hang of it. You'll be best off getting smaller jars—pints and smaller. I have never actually processed anything in a quart jar; all the recipes I've encountered so far are for pints and half pints. Quarter pints are great for jams and sweet preserves. Be a smart shopper and source your jars used from Craigslist, estate sales, garage sales, and the network of grandmas looking to unload their stash. A good friend of mine knows

I'm in a canning craze and snagged a full box of pint and quart jars for me for free from a woman who was getting rid of them.

Buy new jars in off- or end-of-season sales from your local Ace hardware store or big-box stores that you don't mind supporting. The canning season is at its peak during summer and fall, so look for jars in late fall. If you go in on large orders of jars with friends, your local hardware store will probably give you a discount; they're not making much of a profit margin on jars to begin with, so they'll appreciate your business.

- **Extra lids.** If you bought your jars used, or you're consistently reusing your own jars (i.e., your friends are good at returning jars after you grant them canned goodies), you'll need a stash of new lids. Don't buy the ones that come with bands (unless you actually need the bands). Your house will soon be overrun with canning bands, and there's no need to add more to the mix. A box of twelve wide-mouth or regular lids will run you between $2 and $4.
- **Canning utensil kit.** You can find a set for less than $12 or buy a jar lifter and canning funnel piecemeal. These are the only essentials in the kit, although the magnetized lid lifter thingy is really handy.
- **Calculator.** I have yet to can anything (besides peaches) in an overabundance scenario.

Word to the Wise

When buying used jars intended for canning, be sure to feel around the rim for chips or cracks, which will prevent your lids from sealing. It's best to use vintage canning jars as bins to stash grains or as décor since they might break during processing.

You're not likely to make full recipes from any of the Ball books or other put-up-the-whole-season's-harvest books. So in the event you're proportionately lessening the recipe . . . it's highly ambitious (for some of us) to assume we can do mental math (correctly, at least) in the midst of following a recipe.

the dirty word in canning: modify

I have a tenuous relationship with recipes, as you know. And canning recipes are, unfortunately, sticklers for precision. But life happens—even in canning. What if you can't find all the ingredients a recipe calls for, or what if it requires an extra trip out after a long work day for a particular spice or the elusive liquid pectin? Contrary to what everyone says, you can actually modify aspects of canning recipes.

Don't confuse this with creating new recipes, which is unsafe unless you're going to spring for an expensive pH meter (not drugstore strips, which are imprecise at best) to test pH levels. When you change certain elements of a written recipe, you must understand that you are altering the pH of the food. After you've done a little extracurricular reading (see the "Resources" section at the end of the chapter), you'll start to understand what makes recipes safe as they're written. Once you understand how a recipe is safe, then you may

Hip Trick

The best way to reduce a recipe is to see how much of the main ingredient you actually have (either by dicing and placing in measuring cups or by measuring weight, however the recipe lists it). Determine a ratio by dividing how much you have by how much it says to use (hint: the number will be a decimal less than 1). Multiply the quantities of each ingredient in the recipe by your answer.

make slight changes to the things that won't affect acidity levels.

For example, the rhubarb vanilla preserves recipe. I started with a rhubarb rose preserves recipe from Linda Ziedrich's book, but I couldn't find fresh rose petals in the middle of April to save my life. I did, however, find dried hibiscus flowers at my co-op. I swapped the two ingredients in equal measure, since I know it's safe to swap a dried ingredient for fresh rose petals. Rhubarb is a high-acid fruit, and I understand the safety factors involved in the swap; whereas, had the main ingredient been figs (which are just on the edge of safe for water bath canning) I would not have ventured to change anything [in this case, I would have not been able to use this recipe]. Don't be reckless with recipes, but know that you're not nailed to the wall. Here are a few tips to develop a better understanding of safe modifications to recipes:

→ Your bible is "Approximate pH of Foods and Food Products." Type this URL into your browser and then print out the PDF that appears: foodscience.caes.uga.edu /extension/documents/FDAapproximate pHoffoodslacf-phs.pdf.

The FDA/University of Georgia Cooperative Extension may update the information, but at least you have a hard copy to stash away. These fantastic Web resources

quick tip for the unaccustomed

I talk about the acidity of foods, but understanding the numbers linked to highly acidic foods can be confusing. A good rule of thumb for not getting tripped up by the pH scale: **the higher the acidity of the food, the lower the number on the pH scale.**

239

tend to disappear and then reappear in new formats, so try Googling the following terms to find similar lists in the event nothing pops up for you:

- *pH values food*
- *pH values of various foods*
- *Food pH*

If you're trying to gauge accuracy (since the inter-webs are territory where anyone could post a list and say it's correct), seek out a standard for something you know, like tomatoes should be listed as a range between 4.3 and 4.9, and judge your source by how they're listed. The variance is due to differences in cultivars (a plum tomato is more acidic than a beefsteak) and varying degrees of ripeness. Compare pH levels of existing ingredients with any substitution ideas you have.

- Never alter ratios of acidifiers like lemon juice, vinegar, and sometimes actual fruit (oranges, lemons, or other high-acid components of a spread). It's better to find an existing, safe recipe that includes the ingredients you have in mind and just alter the spices and herbs. Also, if a recipe calls for bottled lemon juice, don't take liberties and use freshly squeezed lemon juice; a specific pH level must be achieved, and it requires the consistent pH of the bottled juice, not the variable pH levels of fresh juice.

- Alter sugar and salt levels as you choose. Sugar and salt do not affect safety or alter pH levels of recipes. You use both of these things to maintain the texture of the fruit or vegetable. Sugar is crucial in the gelling process;

240

if you're set on reducing or using alternative sweeteners (like honey or agave nectar), Pomona's Universal Pectin is my fave commercial pectin to have on hand.

- Switch up spices and add dried ingredients (such as fruits and nuts) to your liking, though adding nuts to a spread will increase the processing time required, since it takes longer for heat to permeate a nut than a tender fruit. Look up similar chutney/conserve recipes (recipes that have similar proportions of those ingredients) to find out safe processing times for anything you alter into a chunkier state. Adding spices and herbs does not affect pickling brine ratios, but if you want the freedom to go wild and create, refrigerator pickles are where you should direct those intentions.

- Make your own pectin instead of relying on a commercial brand (which may or may not be readily available to you). Pectin has nothing to do with safety, just aesthetics.

- I'm a big advocate for reducing recipes to accommodate quantities of what you actually have, but you should never double a sweet spread recipe. Just make two batches if you have that much produce. Most sweet spreads won't set properly if there's too much in the pan.

troubleshooting and tips for first-timers

All the things I wish someone would've told me!

General tips and issues:

- When reducing quantities in a recipe, calculate and record new amounts *before* you start prepping and cooking the fruit.

- Wear comfortable shoes throughout the canning/preserving process, out of kindness to your legs. For certain types of spreads or recipes you might be hovering around the pot waiting for the miraculous gel for thirty minutes. I've never completed a start-to-finish canning operation in less than two hours; that's a long time to be standing on a hard floor.

- Timing is more important with some recipes than others. Read through the whole recipe many times to see where you may end up spending more time, and adjust your approach accordingly. If possible, prep the fruits or vegetables way in advance and refrigerate to split up back-to-back stages of prepping, cooking, and then processing.

- Have something clean you can place your utensils or funnel on while you're putting the food in jars. Sometimes it seems like you need five hands in the heat of canning, and an extra plate can do wonders for your sanity. No need to sterilize it; during processing you'll be boiling out any airborne or potential spoilers hiding on the surface.

- Wear your industrial-strength Casabella dish gloves (the ones you bought after reading Chapter 1) from the moment you drop jars in the canner for sterilization to the point when you're removing processed jars of food. They allow you to grab a jar that's marginally attached to the jar lifter or just serve as a buffer from the splashy rolling boil of the water. I don't suggest reaching directly into the water with your gloves though. Even water-stop gloves can't stand up against 8–10 inches of boiling water.

The *Ball Complete Guide to Home Preserving* book has a good problem-solving section, but here are a few things that eluded me or gave me a hard time as I began my canning adventure.
For water bath canning:

- If you have trouble finding sterilized bands in your canner pot or discover the pain-in-the-ass scenario where bands slide beneath your rack during sterilization, try tying bands together loosely with kitchen twine or using a small metal colander to hold bands and submerging the lot in the canner pot.
- When recipes recommend waiting five minutes to pull your jars out of the canner after the required processing time, it's only for you; it doesn't have anything to do with safety of the food, just your arms. And if you'll be processing more jars and don't want to turn off the heat, it's fine to just pluck the jars out of the boiling water carefully.
- Towels at the bottom of your rackless pot might actually hinder your processing time. Consider one of the ideas for a DIY canning rack.

243

Issues with sweet preserves:

- I gave up on myself when it comes to skimming foam gracefully; it always slides right off the spoon. (Maybe I have an elbow malfunction?) Eugenia Bone demonstrated as we both stood in her kitchen that it just takes patience and persistence; keep at it with a broad metal cooking spoon.
- The spoon test (dipping a spoon you've placed in your freezer to test jelly/jam sets) remained elusive to me until I realized that all the syrup is going to slide off the frozen spoon; it's the *last two* drops I should be looking at. They should linger together on the long side of the spoon, which supposedly looks like a sheet to someone (not me). I realized my concord grape jellies had both set after I puzzled over two purple drops clinging to my frozen tablespoon.
- For jams and preserves, an easier plan is to look for changes in the bubbles that alert you to gelling (they become larger and darker). Linda Ziedrich's *The Joy of Jams, Jellies and Other Sweet Preserves* book gives pretty accurate times for when gelling should occur. And remember, if you've reduced a recipe, it will likely gel faster.

For pickles:

- Vegetables bobbing out of the vinegar solution (near the top of jar) is unnerving but not unsafe. Invert and gently shake the contents every so often (after the first day) to redistribute the vinegar.

resources

books

- *Ball Complete Book of Home Preserving* by Judi Kingry and Lauren Devine.

  I use this book mostly to dredge up ideas for ingredients I have on hand, and to understand what recipe combinations are safe. The recipes feel a little mechanical when followed directly since they don't tell you why you do things. After reading other books, though, you'll appreciate this one for what it has: lots of recipes!

- *Canning and Preserving*, in the Homemade Living series, by Ashley English.

  Excellent pictures of the often-confusing things involved in canning. I especially love the photos of each of the various kinds of sweet preserves since there are so many to keep track of!

- *On Food and Cooking* by Harold McGee.

  For all the food and chemistry geeks out there, you must own this book. It's a constant reference that I use to understand why food behaves in certain manners, the historical origins of foods, and how to store foods successfully.

- *The Joy of Pickling* and *The Joy of Jams, Jellies and Other Sweet Preserves* by Linda Ziedrich.

  My go-tos for a food-centered approach to canning. She helps you understand why certain foods are safe to put up and how to play up flavors (not just follow a recipe).

- *Well-Preserved* by Eugenia Bone.

  I wish I could insert the first forty-five pages of Eugenia Bone's book Well-Preserved *directly into this chapter. It's a smart, practical introduction to canning and preserving that would benefit any hip newbie both for canning and for the kitchen at large. Read all the introduction sections, even if you think you won't be curing and smoking meats; there are extremely helpful bits of science behind food and food safety discussed with each type of preservation.*

web

→ foodinjars.com
Get hooked in with the canning blog scene through Marisa's excellent website.

→ csrees.usda.gov/extension
Find your closest cooperative extension office for canning classes, food science/safety questions, and general information.

→ uga.edu/nchfp
The National Center for Home Food Preservation is an excellent resource on all types of food storage and hosts a free, self-paced online course for canning.

→ canningusa.com
Watch the nifty videos featured on this site.

→ foodsafety.psu.edu/preserve.html
Another great place to search for questions that arise with home food preservation. This one is hosted by Penn State.

→ web1.msue.msu.edu/imp/mod01/master01.html
A great database from the Michigan State University Extension Office on preserving food safely.

chapter 10

entertaining projects

test your work

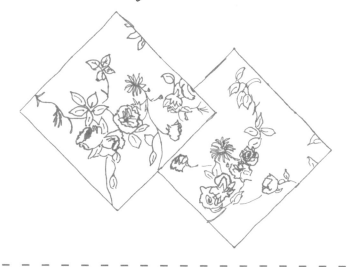

You've worked your way diligently through nine chapters, picked up a bunch of Hip Tricks, and are all the wiser for it. Your efforts in creative problem solving in every area of the house deserve to be shown off. You're now ready for what is hands-down the most fun part of housekeeping: parties!

Get people into your home to eat together and to share and enjoy your space. The happy home is all about momentum, so invite all your nearest and dearest, pronto.

Good reasons to invite people over:

- **Showing off.** It's okay, I give you permission to enjoy showing off. When you work hard at making your house homey, people notice. You can be humble in response to compliments, but always accept praise.
- **Incentive to clean.** I (usually) clean when guests are coming over. The more you invite people over, the more you clean. The more you clean, the less of a burden it becomes.
- **Small gatherings are fun and are cheaper for everyone involved** (as opposed to going out for drinks at a bar). At one of our recent dinner parties we fed eight people, appetizers and desserts included, for $70. You can't even get a sandwich in some places for $9.
- **You'll get invited to parties.** It's infectious amongst friends. Once you host one, your friends will probably reciprocate.

As you've possibly gleaned from reading the rest of the chapters in this book, I'm all for relaxing about everything, and fancying things up as you're ready (or not, if you don't really care). No one is going to judge you by the napkins at your dinner party. If they do, you don't want to be friends with them anyway.

I'm just saying, don't forgo the dinner party because you have a small apartment or only five plates. You've spent enough time with this book to know that simple, cost-effective solutions to home problems are usually just a matter of stopping for a few moments to think it through.

Even people who do special events planning as their profession (like I used to) will assume the harried frenzy of working through hosting preparations. The goal is to have ambiance, comfort, and style in mind at the outset. As the party careens into being, attachments to fancy will start to fade and the focus will become providing a chair, fork, and plate to everyone, pretty cloth napkins optional. Flexibility is the single most important characteristic to acquire as a host; what once seemed so important might need to take a backseat to other practical considerations.

I'll shed some light on the basics of opening your house up to others. There are three kinds of entertaining I'll cover here, each increasing gradually in terms of planning and complexity:

1. Happy houseguests
2. Pimped-out personal parties (dinner or tea parties)
3. Savvy skill-sharing parties (canning, sewing, soap making, silkscreening, yodeling, whatever)

Go forth and celebrate! Be proud of your house—you deserve it. We'll wrap up the chapter with a few essential things to take away after you close this book so you'll be prepared for any situation you encounter in real life.

houseguests in your happy home

Having friends and family stay at your house may conjure a number of different emotions, ranging from genuine excitement to loathing and dread.

Houseguest hip list:

- ❧ Master the art of welcoming someone without waiting on them. There's a fine balance between being welcoming and giving off wait-staff vibes. Show your guests where things are so they can help themselves and feel right at home.
- ❧ Prepare your guests' bed in advance, if possible. It shows that you thought about them and took a few extra minutes ahead of their arrival to make them feel welcome.
- ❧ Make (and eat) breakfast. Since you already do sit-down breakfast (Chapter 8 rubbed off on you, wink, wink), it's not hard to add a coffee cup and seat at the table for your houseguest.
- ❧ Have a spare key so guests can come and go as they please.
- ❧ Relax.

In most cases, you're not obliged to hang with them 24/7 (in-laws may be the exception here). Give yourself some space and let them do their own thing.

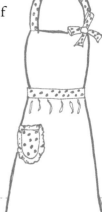

personal parties

Hosting intimate gatherings, small dinner parties, and events like book club or a little cocktail party is not as hard as you might think. You'll do some work on the front end, but then your only job is to enjoy your company and accept praise for how cool your house is. The more you host these kinds of things, the easier it becomes. The learning curve is steep at first, but with time you can crank out a thoughtfully planned party in a few hours.

Entertaining hip list:

- ↦ Give a heads-up with a save-the-date notice. A simple email will suffice to help people block out time for your event on their calendars. Send another email a week before the event with your address, any reminders for things to bring, and other specifics not included in the save-the-date message.
- ↦ Use real dishes. Hit up the thrift store for an extra stash of flatware and plates to pull out on party occasions.
- ↦ Have enough chairs for everyone or remove chairs altogether.
- ↦ Utilize self-serve as often as possible or appropriate.

   The snack and drink station is my favorite way to put guests to the task of making themselves feel welcome. If you're not going to be nearby, you can always make a little tent note (by folding over an index card) saying, "Ice is in the freezer, help yourself!"
- ↦ Who needs matching cups anyway? Your diverse thrift store assortment adds character to the party and makes it easier for guests to remember which cup is theirs.

Hip Trick

Turn a flat of canning jars into perfect party cups. Guests can Sharpie their names onto half-pint or pint-sized mason jars (to keep track of whose glass belongs to whom). As you learned in Chapter 1, you can remove the writing the next day with a swab of rubbing alcohol and then promptly fill the jars with homemade jam.

251

Host the party with another person. That person might be your spouse, best friend, upstairs neighbor, whomever. Just be sure that you have someone else to help with cooking or planning (whichever you don't do the best). I'm the special projects coordinator at my house, so my girlfriend always steps up with the main course, and I've got a pie, homemade ice cream, or some other sweet treat up my sleeve.

For inspiring and crowd-pleasing dishes to serve at dinner parties, please consult my friends Zora O'Neill and Tamara Reynolds. Their book *Forking Fantastic!: Put the Party Back in Dinner Party* is everything it claims to be and will keep you laughing as you follow their crowd-pleasing recipes.

logistics:
it's all in the details

Table. This is the pivotal point of any gathering. If you're not sitting directly at it, then the food is lined up on it, and people will stand around it like a campfire all evening. Revisit Chapter 7 for creative ways to make a couple smaller tables into a larger one. Of the many sit-down gatherings we've hosted in our 800-square-foot apartment, never once

Word to the Wise

Exercise a bit of potluck common sense and be sure to query (or assign) guests on what they plan to bring. Leaving things up in the air can leave you with eight bowls of salsa and no salad or dessert. As potluck host, usually you'll provide the main dish, but it's flexible. In the case of BBQ potlucks you can ask guests to bring their grillables. Getting a feel for what's coming can help make the feast a success.

have my guests noticed a sneaky plank of plywood hiding out underneath the tablecloth. One day I'll have a luxurious, extendable dining room table (and a dining room), but for now it's fun to be creative with what I've got.

◆▸ **Chairs.** Borrow as many as you can from your neighbors. Definitely decline if they have fancy upholstered chairs that might serve as magnets for wine or food (you don't want to spend the next day taking a chair to the dry cleaners). We like to pick up chairs from garage sales and the roadside whenever we see good ones. You can always buy a folding set to have on hand for when dinner expands into a jolly good time.

If you have enough chairs, why not make it a sit-down kind of thing? If you don't have enough chairs, it's totally fine to let guests grab a plate of food and find spots around the house. Lining up available chairs in advance and positioning them in a comfortable conversation shape (a crescent or slight curve so guests can chat) helps with the flow of getting food, sitting down, and eating it.

◆▸ **Linen and swag.** Buy that vinyl Christmas-print tablecloth that's on sale at the flea market or thrift store. I know it's cheesy, but it never hurts to give your tabletop an extra layer of protection. Throw on a pretty tablecloth to hide Santa or display that vinyl number outright at craft parties; getting soap base off the vinyl will be much easier than getting it off cloth.

253

Owning a dark-colored dinner party tablecloth will make you feel like a genius every time you do laundry after a dinner party. I found mine at the thrift store for $4; it's a long, deep purple banquet tablecloth.

Wash (or have ready) all plates, cups, and flatware the night before so you can spend your time the day of the party doing other things around the house.

➻ **Test.** Try sitting at every seat around your makeshift table so you know what each person will see and feel. Maybe you'll need to shift a setting a bit to the left since guests have knees they'll probably want to put under the table.

➻ **Plan.** Having a play-by-play action plan is usually not necessary in informal dinner gatherings you'll host, but knowing that you're going to need to do some dishes in order for guests to have a clean dessert plate is important not to overlook. Zora and Tamara hire a dishwasher for their Sunday night dinners to take the stress off the hosts and keep the clean dishes coming; the money that guests contribute for food goes toward the cost of hiring someone for the evening. Usually at smaller gatherings, a pal will step up in the break between dinner and dessert and offer to do some dishes, to which my response is always, "I'll dry!"

Word to the Wise

Set the table way in advance (like the night before). This is my favorite part of entertaining because I get to pull out all my pretty scavenged cups, napkins, and plates. Or if this isn't your bag, then forget about it. Have guests help you set the table to keep them occupied before it's time to eat.

how to set the table

For sit-down civilized dinner, the simplest version goes like this: Napkin on left, fork on napkin. Plate in center. Knife blade facing the plate on the right side of the setting. I've always needed to check because I could never remember. *The Joy of Cooking* has more elegant alternatives should you need them, like for two-fork occasions, and can tell you what the hell to do with a dessert spoon (though there's no input given on where to find room on your makeshift table for a fancy table setting).

The strategic placement of linens makes things seem more official. I like to demarcate the beverage station with a pretty blue tea towel, sometimes placing cups there and other times using it to house tea pitchers or wine bottles. (Since you aced Chapter 6, you now know how to remove any wine dribbles in the event any of your linens get spotted.)

assignments on arrival

The first guests to arrive get assignments at my house. The first person gets set up on drinks and assigned as beverage coordinator. The second person to arrive becomes designated door answerer and greeter. The two people get to know each other (if they don't already), and your arriving guests are managed smoothly. You can continue to run around in a frenzy and attempt to look calm.

hip trick

Ever sit down at a tightly set table and wonder which drinking glass is yours? A sassy friend once showed me how to tell. Make night-vision glasses with the thumbs and forefingers of both hands; your left hand forms a lowercase *b* (for bread) and your right hand forms a lowercase *d* (for drink). Never leave home without your thumbs.

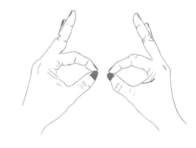

You'll have more fun with it if you forget any preconceived notions of what a dinner party should be like. The most successful party is not based on fancy food, décor, matching chairs, or other crap. Nope, dinner party success is solely based on friends sitting around talking together over food you made.

craft and knowledge-share parties

Hosting skill share parties is a great way to get people in your house and learn something new and handy while you're at it. All skill share parties have a few things in common:

- **Plan/host it with at least one person who actually knows the craft/skill** in question (if you don't already know how to do it yourself).
- **Location, location, location.** Said person who knows what he or she is doing will be crucial in determining if your house will work well for the proposed activity. If the party requires a lot of counter space and your countertop is the size of a small cutting board, don't despair, just talk to your pals about possibly using their houses. Your pad might work for a sewing party where guests use their laps as workspace.
- You'll need to either provide **supplies** for everyone or provide a supply list that guests must bring in order to participate. Assigning one or two people to supplies acquisition and then having guests pay their share is a good way to split the costs collectively and avoid logistical mayhem.

- **Snacks and beverages** are always a good idea. Swing it potluck or BYOB style, or ask guests to chip in a couple of dollars to cover you at the grocery or liquor store.

Craft and knowledge-share parties can be any size, from bigger, organized ordeals to small, impromptu gatherings. Remember, even one or two friends (and their knitting needles) can make it a party.

Here are a few ideas for parties to get you started, or simply build a party around anything that you've been itching to learn—maybe silk screening, pasta making, or bread baking. Or just revive the stitch-and-bitch gathering by offering to host.

soap party

Last fall, my friends Liz, Adriana, and I hosted a soap party at my house where we learned (via Liz) and practiced the melt and pour soap-making method. We each brought and shared things to jazz up our soap, like essential oils, spices such as turmeric and paprika for color, and dried flowers and pretty herbs for character. A share of the soap base ended up costing $7 per person, which sufficed to make a huge stash of handmade presents for everyone on our holiday shopping lists. Counter space and access to a few burners on the stovetop is a must for this party.

Word to the Wise

In the case of splitting supply costs among attendees, let guests know when they RSVP that they will still be responsible for their share of the costs if they flake or cancel at the last minute. In some cities or circles this won't be an issue at all, but in other places it's good to let people know ahead of time so that you or the rest of the guests don't get stuck covering the cost.

sewing party

I hosted a sewing party at my friend (and brilliant seamstress) Briana's house. Attendees were of all different skill levels, from I've-never-dared-step-so-close-to-a-sewing-machine to yeah-I'll-add-ruffles-to-that-no-biggie. I'm definitely in the former category, so the collective vibes from a group of ladies knocking out mending and tackling creative fabric projects was just what I needed to inspire me. I brought over a bunch of homemade goodies (to keep costs low) and wine and asked guests to chip in $10 to cover those costs plus Briana's time in teaching many of us the ropes on her sewing machine.

This is a great party to host in smaller apartments because guests are (for the most part) stationed in one spot and don't need much space beyond the occasional floor or bed for folding or cutting fabric.

canning party

This fall I hosted a canning party in conjunction with the Canning Across America collective's Canvolution weekend, where home canners participate in a weekend of putting food up collectively spanning all areas of the country. I enlisted my favorite East Coast preserver ladies—Audra from the blog *Doris and Jilly Cook* and Marisa from the *Food in Jars* blog—and the three of us hosted our favorite recipes and acquired the requisite supplies and ingredients. There were ten of us in total, skill levels ranging from newbies to old hats. At the end of the day we split the costs, each paying $10 for a share of the supplies, and everyone went home with two pint jars of pickled green beans, a half pint of peach chutney, a quarter pint of plum lemon jam, and a quarter pint of ketchup.

You don't have to invite famous people over in order to host a kick-ass canning party; it's just a fun way to share what you've learned in the kitchen with friends. Everyone helps with the work and then everyone goes home with tasty foods in jars. If it's going to be more than just a few of you, you'll need a big enough kitchen, with ample counter space and plenty of cooling and ventilation, since all four burners will be going at once.

collage party

A few years ago I got the idea to invite people over to tear up magazines and fun fancy paper (which I always seem to have an excess of), share glue sticks, and drink tea. I came up with the collage and tea party idea because it seemed like a shame that no one had time for creativity in the hustle and bustle of everyday life. It was cool to see friends who swear by the motto "I'm not creative" with their tongues out, poised in concentration, over a no-pressure collage. I fit eight people (and their respective eight floor fans of torn scraps) into my apartment's tiny living room. (Sometimes moving furniture out of the living room is the best way to open your small space to guests.)

I was bummed when the group outgrew my house, though of course delighted that more people were keen on the slow art of glue sticks. But my local library offered free use of their meeting rooms (when planned way in advance). We just made sure to clean up all the little scraps that are inevitable in a paper massacre party.

host a food swap

Food swaps are a great way to diversify your pantry while getting to know your neighbors and fellow make-it-yourself community. Our group trades swappable items like loaves of bread, jars of preserves, backyard-chicken eggs, portions of soup, packages of homemade candy, and the like.

Set up your swap rules however you please. We decided to keep things simple and only stick with food items that *YOU* made (not the farmers' market jam mistresses, not the local artisan baker, etc.). [There are larger share groups called time banks that exist for members to swap services, skills, and sometimes goods. Check the resources section at the end of the chapter to learn more about these groups or to find one in your area.]

Arrange for attendees to bring a homemade potluck item in addition to their swap goods so there will be snacks, and you're not put out to feed and entertain 20 people. Food people like to bring food to events, trust me. Everyone wants to show off something they took the time to prepare. Adding a potluck feature also opens the event to people who maybe don't have a swap item, but would like to join in the food fun with a group of like-minded friends.

the take-away

Keep learning, hip people! Beginners, I promise you, if you keep with it, there's nothing that won't become normal in your house.

The nature of this project has kept me on my toes for the past year. With every new skill I picked up (including second, third, tenth attempts doing things) I began to realize that everything I want to say is not possibly going to fit into a single book. There are always new things to learn and new and better ways of doing things. It all boils down to the wise words of Eleanor Roosevelt: *You must do the thing you think you cannot do.*

Here's a short list of things to take with you into the homemaking endeavors that intimidate you the most:

- **Approach the project with confidence.** Your attitude is likely the single most inhibiting factor in the success of whatever you're attempting to accomplish. Choosing to succeed does wonders. Of course failure will still happen, but at least you're not gearing toward it from the onset.
- **Find mentors.** Follow in the footsteps of people who know more than you and whom you admire. Take time to actually read their books (or blogs) and remember that even they started somewhere.
- **Take stock.** Stop every now and then to appreciate the view from where you've climbed. When I grumble about the loads of extra dishes that accumulate after ice cream or bread making, I take a minute to look around at my kitchen or gawk inside my fridge at the jars of homemade goodies. I remember that not so long ago none of this stuff existed in my house. And I never fail to swell with secret pride when I offer guests a bowl of homemade ice cream. It feels good to say, "I made this." Enjoy it.
- **Teach someone else.** Via the Internet, your kitchen, or while in line at the hardware store. We all inspire each other in different ways. Showing someone the

art of thrift shopping, compost piling, or fridge pickling could unlock the home front for someone else. Two happy homies in their homes now, instead of one.

➻ **Give yourself a break.** You're human. There is no such thing as perfect. Your best effort is always good enough. Putting your feet up and ignoring [insert task-at-hand here] is sometimes what has to be done. Give it your best, and if necessary, try again tomorrow.

resources

books

➻ *Forking Fantastic!: Put the Party Back in Dinner Party* by Zora O'Neill and Tamara Reynolds.
These ladies will crack you up and remind you not to worry about silly details. Dinner parties are supposed to be about food and friends, not napkins.

➻ *The Joy of Cooking* (any edition).
Great illustrations of where things go on the table should you decide to up the fancy ante.

➻ *The Sharing Solution: How to Save Money, Simplify Your Life & Build Community* by Janelle Orsi and Emily Doskow.
Great ideas and resources for planning a meal share or pot-luck event.

➻ *Put 'Em Up: A Comprehensive Home Preserving Guide for the Creative Cook* by Sherri Brooks Vinton.

She has a great little section about working in groups on canning projects, complete with task lists for different types of recipes.

web

➥ timebanks.org
Join (or start) a time bank, an unconventional way to barter and share skills with people in your community.

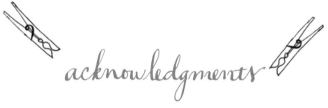

acknowledgments

It truly takes a village to write a comprehensive, no-fear homemaking guide. I couldn't have done it without expert advice from Kate Bussmann, Brianna Campbell, Liz Neves, Gail Maurer and John Neves, Audra Wolfe, Marisa McClellan, Kat Selvocki, Chris Musser, Ulla Kjarval, Andy Roberts and Michelle Diaz, Jen Marine, Wanalee Romero, Jonah Safer, Cassie Hager, Elio Schaechter, Aaron Zimmerman, and everyone at the New York Writers Coalition.

Thank you to friends Zora O'Neill and Tamara Reynolds for the advice, support, and excellent food throughout the book process. A special thank you to Eugenia Bone for welcoming me into your home and offering constant guidance and keen revisions on the food chapters.

Thank you to everyone who made this book happen.

My super-smart and sharp editor at HarperCollins, Julia Abramoff.

My crazy-talented illustrator and agent, Meredith Dawson.

My wonderful pen pal and calligraphy goddess, Alison Hanks.

All of you helped to make this book the most beautiful and artful book I could possibly imagine.

I owe my mom everything for all the years it wasn't easy, when money was tight and time was hard to come by. You made it look easy. Thank you for teaching me how to clean with vinegar and for reading my blog regularly (and being my biggest fan). Thank you to my dad and brother, and to my grandmas Mannie and Jinny. I love you all.

Most important, I'm eternally grateful for my partner, my best friend, my wife-to-be, Jo Ann Santangelo. Without your support, love, all the amazing dinners you cook for us (and, of course, your photographs!), this project wouldn't even exist. Making a home with you is everything I've ever dreamed of.